PEOPLE ARE TALKING ABOUT LEAN FOR LIFE!

"I was self-conscious, fat, and fed up. I vowed to myself that I would do the program 100%—and I did. In five months, I lost more than 40 pounds!"

— *Margaret Kelman, 47*
Lost 50 pounds

"I lost 100 pounds in just ten months. My greatest thrill was hearing my seven-year-old granddaughter say, 'Gee, Grandma, now I can put my arms all the way around you.'"

— *June M. Griesemer, 69*
Lost 115 pounds

"Lean for Life is the only program I've ever tried where I didn't feel hungry."

— *John Morgan, 43*
Lost 63 pounds

"I'm an orchestra conductor, and the compliments and congratulations I've gotten since losing 90 pounds are music to my ears. But more important than how I look is how I feel—I have more energy than ever!"

— *Elizabeth Wright, 23*
Lost 90 pounds

"Before I became Lean for Life, I was too slow to try out for sports. But the program helped me lose weight, learn to eat right, build up my confidence, and get me in shape for football."

— *Eric Eastman, 13*
Lost 45 pounds

"This phenomenal program has given me back my life! I'm so grateful I found it."

— *Susan Gardanier, 37*
Lost 85 pounds

"I'm a baker and I love to eat, but I realized things had to change the day I tipped the scales at 299 pounds. I lost 106 pounds in eight months—and feel better than I ever have."

— *Vince Pilato, 36*
Lost 106 pounds

"The principles I've learned on the program have instilled a sense of discipline and focus—not only in the way I eat, but in my business life as well. Once I made up my mind to go for it, the process was painless."

— *Tim Klein, 49*
Lost 77 pounds

"I think different, I act different, and I look different. Lean for Life has changed my life. It works!"

— *Princess Leali, 34*
Lost 100 pounds

Also by Cynthia Stamper Graff

Lean for Life Phase Two: Lifetime Solutions

bodyPRIDE
(with Janet Eastman and Mark C. Smith)

Lean for Life®

PHASE ONE
WEIGHT LOSS

SECOND EDITION

CYNTHIA STAMPER GRAFF
WITH JERRY HOLDERMAN

Foreword by
PETER VASH, M.D., M.P.H.
Assistant Clinical Professor, UCLA School of Medicine
Past President, American Society of Bariatric Physicians
Executive Medical Director, Lindora Medical Clinics

Griffin Publishing Group

LIBRARY OF CONGRESS CATALOGING-IN-PUBLICATION DATA

Stamper Graff, Cynthia.
Lean for Life Phase One: Weight Loss / by Cynthia Stamper Graff with Jerry Holderman.
1. Diet. 2. Weight Loss. 3. Health. 4. Fitness.
5. Nutrition. I. Jerry Holderman. II. Title.

ISBN 58000-088-6

Second Edition
Printed in the United States of America

10 9 8 7 6 5 4 3 2 1

This book is in no way intended to be a substitute for the medical advice of a personal physician. We advise and encourage the reader to consult his/her physician before beginning this or any other weight management and/or exercise program. The authors and the publisher disclaim any liability or loss, personal or otherwise, resulting from the procedures in this book.

An important part of any effort to improve your health is the decision to seek and use help from trusted health professionals from the very start. MENTORS Daily Mental Training is not intended as a substitute for such help, and the authors and manufacturers of MENTORS Daily Mental Training materials and programs disclaim all liability for any injury or illness sustained in connection with their use.

To my parents,

Marshall and Nell Stamper

TABLE OF CONTENTS

ACKNOWLEDGMENTS

Cynthia Stamper Graff

This book wouldn't exist if it weren't for two very special families—the Stamper family and the Lindora family. I am blessed to be a member of both.

My father and mother, Marshall and Nell Stamper, are also the parents of Lindora. They raised both of us on fundamental principles of positive expectation. I will always be grateful to them for believing in me and trusting that I could and would make appropriate "life choices." I am honored to share with others some of the wisdom I have learned from them.

I also thank my daughter Ali, who always understood that while "Mommy's book" was very important, it was never more important than she is.

The loving support of my brothers, Steve Stamper and Bernie Stamper, my sister Kitty Nordstrom, and their families also means a great deal to me. I appreciate their bearing with me during the writing of this book, especially when I seemed "preoccupied" at family functions.

The Lindora family has been equally supportive. Special thanks to:

Peter Vash, M.D., M.P.H., who was always accessible and wise with his input. Our Friday brainstorming sessions are consistently a highlight of my week, and the ideas generated during those working lunches continue to improve the program in very significant ways.

Jan Hunter, R.N., who was truly a treasured resource during her 17 years with Lindora.

Leslie Wulff, R.N, Vice President, Clinic Operations, who blends her strong business skills and a determined commitment to those we serve in ways that benefit thousands of Lindora patients every day.

Debbie Riley, L.V.N., Lindora's Nurse Educator, who has been tireless in her efforts to ensure that this book addressed the everyday problems our patients encounter. In addition to her superb teaching skills, Debbie is a master at moderating chats, hosting online forums, and providing other support tools to our atHome and Lean for Life Online clients.

Joe Risser, M.D., M.P.H., who is a sensitive, caring physician. He also happens to be a techno-wizard. I can always count on his thorough research and thoughtful analysis, and I appreciate both very much.

Keith McGuinness, whose passion for making the Lean for Life program available to people throughout the world via the Internet has been a vital contribution not only to our company, but to the lives of the many thousands of people who visit www.leanforlife.com every day.

Thank you, as well, to Andral Dugger, M.D., Judi Goldstone, M.D., Lynne Nieto, N.P., Cay Taylor, N.P., Patricia O'Donnell, N.P., and Jeanette Schmidt, N.P. for their service to Lindora and the care they consistently show our patients, as well to Jackie Martinez, L.V.N., Jackie Rosen, R.N., Jayme Davidson, R.N., Brenda Parks, R.N., Ryan Mariden, Dollie Tenorio, L.V.N., and Sherrie Theckston, for their ongoing efforts to constantly improve the Lindora program and those who administer it.

Kathy Walker, R.N. Carol Mulvey, L.V.N., and Team Orange inspired the original "atHome" patients to make the lifestyle changes necessary for achieving lasting weight control. Their successful approach in reaching out to people unable to visit our clinics demonstrated that the principles of our program can truly work for anyone, anywhere. The motivating messages sent by Melanie Dingle, L.V.N., to our atHome clients never cease to warm my heart or inspire success in those who receive them.

I appreciate every member of Lindora's corporate team, whose commitment to helping people become Lean for Life was apparent every time they pulled together to support me when it seemed like I had three full-time jobs. First, to my capable and always intuitive assistant, Billye Littman, thank you for all you do for me. I also greatly appreciate the contributions of our first class corporate team, including Stella Gates, Donna Rockenbach, Mike Quinn, Karen TerBorg, Al Andres, Jeff Beltz, Adam Cham, Todd Cornish, Vince Duong, Kristina Gerke, Christine Gil, Danielle Gray, John Hendricks, Rauha Hilander, Leon Lombardo, Dalonda Mahoney, Olivia Moreno, Gustavo Rivera, Patti Sewell, James Scott, Bert Smith, Thao Tran, Katherine Trueblood, Joe Walton, Georgia Weichel, Corinne Wikle, Mark Wisniewski, and Stacie Yee.

Team Lindora is comprised of the hundreds of women and men whose commitment to promoting good health and longevity makes a difference in the lives of many people every day. Without each of them, this book would not be what it is. They not only encouraged me with cards and calls, but encouraged their patients to share their stories so that others could benefit from their experiences. Special thanks to the following who have contributed to Lindora's success through their many years of service: Rita Martinez, Terry Chronister, Carlene Brown, Emily VanderWoude, Cynthia Morelos, Vickie Flatt, Evelyn Lichten, Pauline Espinoza-Garcia, Heather Ferber, Angela Major, Cathy Markuson, Paola Martinez, Krista Jarrard, Shirley Joratz, Jane Warner, Kay Bennett, Kathy Sandstrum, Francie Gendusa, Cynthia Encinas, Shirley Prather, Teresa Brady, Jan Forde, Janet Lynch, Jeanette Bader-Frijas, Gayle Udolph, Tiffany Robertson, Audrey Smith, Treena Totin-Limon, Cheryl Turner, Jennifer Macofsky, Peggy DeWitt, Alisa Blansett, Lori Spencer, Annette Minicucci, Meg

Whittington, Beatrice Sorotsky, Audrey Chironis-Grant, Wendy Henderson, Patricia Iacono, Sandra Delella, Tammi Coulombe, Sandra Hulsey, Deborah Tullio, Vickie Dilag, Rebecca Sanchez, Barb Mariani, Carol Vega-Aguilar, Andrea Taylor, Julie Zehra-London, Veronica Razo, Vicki Lawson, Lyliane Cheneau, Leticia Gaviola, Sherry Killingsworth, Elaine Wilt, Suzanne Bowman, Stephanie North, Jean Kennedy, Marinette Dacumos, Lupe Nunez, Arlene Medina, Deborah Sozzani, Paula Manriquez, Marcia Knott, Cheryl Lewis, Janet Coleman, Mary Maddock, Carol McGuinnis, Julie Cohen, Kathleen Shaw, Carole Bass, Florence Buchanan, Kathleen Christianson, Maria Castro, Ann Hoang, Jeannie Arciniega, Melinda Hunziker, Maria Arkoncel, and Melanie Batanga.

Mike and Kim Kollen's excellent work on creating and refining the Lean for Life website is truly appreciated. Eric Flamholtz and Yvonne Randle at Management Systems have helped Lindora become a stronger organization. The business disciplines they've helped us develop have strengthened the organization; this book is a result of the strategic planning we did together.

To my fellow YPO'ers, I thank you all—especially the members of my forum (you know who you are!). I constantly learn from each of you and from the "resources" available to us.

There are several people whose contributions in the field of obesity research have been especially meaningful to me. Thank you to Issie Greenberg, Ph.D. and George Blackburn, M.D. for the always outstanding Harvard Obesity Conferences. Every one has proven valuable in helping us further refine our program, and Dr. Blackburn's words of encouragement many years ago contributed to Lindora's strong commitment to research data collection. Steven Phinney, M.D., Ph.D., and Dennis Jones, Ph.D. have conducted significant research that validates the efficacy and safety of ketosis in the dieting state; Tom Wadden, Ph.D., professor of psychology at the University of Pennsylvania School of Medicine, has provided encouragement and positive feedback about our program and has motivated me personally with his wonderful lectures on behavior modification and the importance of ongoing maintenance.

I want to acknowledge and thank Steven Blair, P.E.D., especially for his Harvard Conference lecture on the efficacy of exercising more often for shorter periods, which helped inspire Lindora's emphasis on movement and moderate exercise. Richard Atkinson , M.D. deserves recognition for his vision in launching the American Obesity Association (AOA) and for his commitment to the compassionate clinical treatment of obesity. The research legacy of George Bray, M.D. has inspired Lindora to strive for improvement in providing unparalleled patient care. And a very special thanks to John Foreyt, Ph.D. at Baylor University. His lectures on behavior modification are always enlightening, and I appreciate his belief in me and his encouragement of the project.

There are two professional organizations that have been enormously important to me personally, as well as to the development of the Lindora program. The research conducted by members of the North American

Association for the Study of Obesity (NAASO) affords Lindora an opportunity to continue being "cutting edge." The American Society of Bariatric Physicians (ASBP) is dedicated to the principles of advancing ethical clinical treatment of the obese patient. Lindora has grown as an organization from the opportunities that ASBP has given us to share our experiences and to learn from other members.

I'm so happy to have collaborated with Harry Wexler, Ph.D., Ellen McGrath, Ph.D., Carol Lindquist, Ph.D., and other colleagues at The Psychology Center in Laguna Beach, California on an extraordinary project involving groundbreaking psychological testing of the overweight and obese. Our association gave me the added momentum to make this book even better when I was convinced I'd given it all I could. I appreciate the friendship and personal support I receive from Harry and Ellen.

Robert Schwartz listened to me talk "content" for hours and was always generous with ideas and material. Heartfelt thanks to Gloria Duboise, whose encouraging cards and notes seemed to always arrive at just the right time, and Estelle Kevitch and Nancy Nevile-Smith, true friends who were always there. I want to acknowledge the creative insight and emotional support I've received from Karen York. Roger Riddell deserves special thanks for always seeking the best ways to market Lindora. I also appreciate Tom Gehring's care and concern.

To Maury Povich and Liz Frillizia, a heartfelt "thank you." This book is, in large part, the result of the intense interest generated in the Lindora program by Diana Rosenfield's and Frieda Nielsen's numerous appearances on Maury's show. I also appreciate the sensitivity that Kathleen Sullivan and staff at Lifetime displayed while sharing Diana's story. And of course, my deepest appreciation goes to Diana Rosenfeld, Tommy McGruder, and Frieda Nielsen, three Lean for Life ambassadors who have motivated thousands by going public with their stories.

Thank you, too, to Janet Eastman and Mark Smith, for their editorial insight; to Frank Groff for his energetic, enterprising work on behalf of Lindora; to Lance Huante and p11 creative for consistently spectacular graphic creations; to Pure Octane for their marketing savvy; to Michael Marcheschi at m2design group for his attention to detail and collaborative spirit; to Mary Grady at KCBS for thinking of Lindora and caring enough about Tommy McGruder to call; to Ashley Gardner at Pandora Productions for always coming through with brilliance and originality on a moment's notice; and to Griffin Publishing Group—especially Bob Howland, Robin Howland, and Bryan Howland—for sharing our enthusiasm and trusting that this wouldn't be "just another diet book."

I'm profoundly grateful to Herman Frankel, M.D., and his partner, Jean Staeheli, of Portland Health Institute. Their collaboration made the whole project more enjoyable and memorable. The energy and ideas that were generated during the days and nights we spent together were gifts that I will always treasure. I am fortunate to have them as my "mental trainers" and personal "BioModifiers." They were there for me 100%, and their warmth and wisdom is reflected throughout this book.

Finally, I want to thank Jerry Holderman, my collaborator and partner on this project. Interest and enthusiasm are essential to accomplish anything of value, and Jerry possesses an abundance of both. Over the years, we've had our share of "special moments." Jerry has been there to prod me along with his wicked wit, always striving to make the finished product the very best it could possibly be. It's so reassuring to know I can always count on him. His unique talent in translating mountains of complex material into the inspiring, highly readable book you're holding is a testament to Jerry's remarkable "way with words."

Jerry Holderman

This book has been a true collaboration from the very beginning, blending the experience, talent, and perspective of dozens of people who were committed to excellence and determined to achieve nothing less.

Cynthia Stamper Graff's vision and passion are evident on every page of this book. Her commitment to creating a finished product that would truly benefit its readers has been unwavering, and her enthusiasm has been unabashed. Her resilience and grace under pressure are gifts. I thank her for believing in this project and in me. My respect for her talent and tenacity has only grown during our collaboration.

I also owe a huge personal debt to five other extraordinary people whose vital contributions have helped make this book what it is:

Debbie Riley, L.V.N.—Her knowledge of the Lean for Life program is unparalleled, and her willingness to share her wisdom and experience has made the process of writing this book—and the book itself—so much more than it might have been. Debbie truly cares about the people who turn to the Lean for Life program for support and success, and her contributions to this book have been significant.

Herman M. Frankel, M.D.—Dozens of times during the writing of the first edition of this book, Dr. Frankel ended our telephone conversations with, "I'm with you all the way!" He absolutely was, and words can't express how much I value his wisdom and friendship. He is the godfather of this project.

Jean Staeheli—Her keen insights and astonishing creative consistency were as invaluable in generating ideas and clarifying concepts as they were in coaxing this manuscript across the finish line. Jean is the consummate team player, and her ability to nurture and elicit from others their best—whether she's listening or speaking—is a unique gift.

Janet Eastman— Her editorial instincts and wit are every bit as sharp—and appreciated—as the day we met 20 years ago. Thank you, Janet.

Terry O'Neill— His emotional intelligence, unique perspective, and extraordinary encouragement make a difference in my life every day.

I'm deeply grateful, as well, for a small but stalwart circle of close friends whose support I treasure: Rick Davis, Veston Rowe, Gary Costa, Kiko Rodriguez, Joyce Pederson, Jack Herzberg, Mary Beth Nelson, Megan Hodges, Ali Fadakar, Rev. Dr. Tari Lennon, Deborah Olson, and Jared Olson-Gomez.

Thank you, too, to my family. No matter where they are, they are with me: Ruth Lawrence, Daniel Holderman, Dorothy Sebell, Leonard Sebell, Kathy Holderman, Jim Holderman, Rachele Daly, Jim Daly, Austin Daly, Judy Eratosene, Zelma Dolph, Harold Dolph, Alice Holderman, Gerald Holderman, Nellie Jackson, and Clara Dutch Spalding.

I also thank Dr. Marshall Stamper for generously sharing his wisdom and his knowledge; Nell Stamper, who elevates Southern hospitality to new heights; Diana Rosenfeld, for sharing her heart and soul and for inspiring so many to do so much; and six other special people whose ongoing commitment to the Lindora program and the people it serves is apparent every time we talk—Peter Vash, M.D., Joe Risser, M.D; Leslie Wulff, R.N., Keith McGuinness, Jayme Davidson, R.N., and Lynne Nieto, N.P.

Thanks to everyone at "Team Lindora," especially to Olivia Beltz, Melanie Dingle, Rauha Hilander, Mike Kollen, Billye Shinto Littman, Sherrie Theckston, Kathy Walker, Stacie Yee, and Georgia Weichel.

Frank Groff helped get the ball rolling—thank you, Frank, for the vote of confidence and for making the connection. Thanks, too to the management at Griffin Publishing Group—Bob Howland, Robin Howland, and Bryan Howland— for seeing the potential of this project and for doing their best to maximize it.

I also value the enormous creative contribution that Lance Huante and the entire crew at p11 creative—especially Dan Webster, Wayne Yong, and Alex Chao—have made the look and feel of the finished product. Their collective sense of taste and style is equaled only by their patience. Michael Marcheschi at m2design group made working on this project during the homestretch a true pleasure.

Many others have also supported me along the way through their words and actions. My thanks to Edward Abraham, M.D., Richard Ammon, Ph.D., Patricia Bell, William J. Bell, Mike Bertsch, Kate Navin Booth, Rev. Dr. Cynthia Cavalcanti, Sandy Davis, Belinda DeLong, Phyllis Ensminger, `Xavier Espinoza, Steven Fisher, Michael Foxworthy, Daniel Franco, Phyllis Frase, Bob Frase, Agnes Griffith, Moana Grochow, Nigel Hampton, Ph.D., Jack Hanson, Dee Dee Hanson, Jim Heinz, Megan Hodges, John Humphrey, Maxine Humphrey, Steve Huston, Carolyn Johnson, Cynthia Juno, Jill Kasofsky, Jeff Kaufman, Ron Kipke, Marc LaFont, Mary Ann Lowe, Jay Marzullo, Norma McCarty, Ellen McGrath, Ph.D., William Nagel, Gary Parsons, Trena Parsons, Rafael Rosario, Manny Rosas, Mark Smith, Gwen Stewart, Duncan Strauss, Joyce Ukropina, Javier Villalobos, Honey Ward, Phoebe Ward, Harry Wexler, Ph.D., and Joanne Winslow.

And, of course, Charlotte, who was there every step of the way.

FOREWORD

by Peter Vash, M.D., M.P.H.
Former President, American Society of Bariatric Physicians
Assistant Clinical Professor, UCLA School of Medicine
Executive Medical Director, Lindora Medical Clinics

Although hundreds of weight loss programs and diet books have come and gone over the past 35 years, Americans today are fatter than ever. Back in 1961, about 25% of the population was obese. Current statistics indicate that more than 60% of the United States adult population is overweight or obese.

This striking increase isn't the result of any alteration in genetic factors. No one's DNA has changed. And while life and the way we live it is unquestionably different from the way it once was, the basic structure of our lives is not. Back then, people had jobs, attended school, played sports, raised kids, and went to the movies. We still do.

What has changed, however, is the way many of us have chosen to react to the rapidly changing, increasingly stressful environment in which we live. While you may not be able to pinpoint exactly why you've gained weight, you can do something to change it. You possess the power to regain your health, dignity, and future, and the support and guidance this book provides can help you do it. You can lose weight. You can learn how to maintain your weight within a safe, healthy range. You can become Lean for Life.

I was first introduced to the Lindora Medical Clinics and the Lean for Life program in 1990, when, as president of the American Society of Bariatric Physicians, I was asked to give a presentation to the company's medical staff. What impressed me most about the people at Lindora was their deep-rooted commitment to the principles of compassionate patient care and the apparent results they were achieving.

When I first reviewed the Lindora program, it struck me as sensible, safe, and effective. It was devoid of hype and supported with solid scientific merit. The program is built upon a medically sound, common-sense foundation. Once you understand and apply its principles, you can be confident in your ability to not only lose your excess fat, but to keep it off.

The weight-loss principles on which the Lean for Life program is based have stood the test of time for more than a quarter-century, helping hundreds of thousands of obese people regain control of their bodies and their lives. The program continues to be just as effective today. Few of the "breakthrough" diets, best-selling diet books, or self-styled diet-and-fitness gurus are around or even remembered after a few years, but Lindora has been and will continue to be.

As Executive Medical Director of Lindora, my responsibility is to bring to the program new scientific advances that will enhance safe and effective weight loss. While the field of obesity treatment continues to be filled with quack remedies and bogus professionals promising miracle cures, the Lean for Life program continues to incorporate only the soundest of scientific principles.

This is a book about change—changing the way you eat, feel, think, look, and live. It's about investing in your own health and happiness. Anyone who uses this book on their weight-loss journey can be assured of having a responsible, reliable guide.

THE LEAN FOR LIFE ADVANTAGE

*"If you always do what you've always done,
you'll always get what you always got."*
—Anne Kaiser Stearns

This is much more than a book about how to lose weight. It's about making changes in the way you eat, the way you look, the way you feel, and the way you think. It features a comprehensive, personalized program based on more than thirty years of clinical research and experience. The Lean for Life program addresses the many physiological, psychological, and environmental factors that cause people to risk their health by being overweight. If you follow this program, you will not only lose weight, you will learn to keep it off.

I know that the process of losing weight can be a challenge. I also know that for many people, *not* losing weight is even more challenging—and definitely more painful. Once you've made the decision to become Lean for Life, this book will help you take action to create positive, healthy changes in your body and your life. *Lean for Life Phase 1: Weight Loss* will guide you through a straightforward, results-oriented program designed to help you lose weight rapidly, safely, and comfortably. One month from today, you can weigh 10 to 15 pounds less than you do right now—and you can repeat the Weight Loss phase of the program until you lose all the weight you want!

The eating plan and success strategies featured in this book have been refined over time. Since 1971, when my father, Marshall Stamper, M.D, opened the first Lindora Medical Clinic, Lindora nurses and doctors have worked exclusively with overweight people, *logging more than ten million patient treatments.* This book presents what we've learned along the way in a daily format that's designed to be easy to follow and fun to do. As you move through the program day by day, I hope you'll experience for yourself how the knowledge, awareness, and skills you gain can support you in becoming—and staying—Lean for Life!

THE TWO-PHASE APPROACH TO BECOMING—AND STAYING—LEAN FOR LIFE

The Lean for Life program is divided into two phases: the Weight Loss/Metabolic Adjustment phase and the Lifetime Maintenance phase. During both phases, you'll be eating healthy, nutritious foods that are readily available at grocery stores and restaurants.

Weight Loss is designed as a 28-day module. During this module, you'll be limiting your calories and your intake of carbohydrates—your body's primary energy source—so that your body will rely on its alternate energy system, excess body fat, for energy. You'll learn more about how this low fat, moderate protein, low carbohydrate nutritional plan can help you achieve a safe and motivating rate of weight loss on pages 19-21.

After each module of Weight Loss, you will move on to Metabolic Adjustment. During this 14-day period, you'll be increasing your body's metabolism—the rate at which you burn calories—by gradually adding selected foods to your eating plan. Metabolic Adjustment is carefully structured to help you retain the results you've achieved during Weight Loss. When you do it properly, you will adjust your metabolism, allowing you to eat larger portions without experiencing a weight gain. If you have more weight to lose, you'll begin another Weight Loss module after completing Metabolic Adjustment.

As anyone who has ever dieted knows, losing weight is only the first step. The challenge is maintaining a healthy weight, which is exactly what the second phase of the program is designed to help you achieve. Once you've lost all the weight you want to lose and have successfully completed Metabolic Adjustment, you'll proceed to "Phase 2: Lifetime Maintenance." During Phase 2, the goal is specific: to adjust your physiologic setpoint to your new leaner weight so that you can begin to appropriately eat a wider variety of foods and more calories without gaining weight.

THE LEAN FOR LIFE PROGRAM OVERVIEW

THE "PREP": 1-3 DAYS

A period of one to three days during which you prepare your body and your mind for "Phase 1: Weight Loss."

WEIGHT LOSS: up to 28 DAYS

After completing the "Prep" days, you will begin the active *Weight Loss* portion of Phase 1, which lasts 28 days (or less, depending on your weight loss goal).

Week 1	Days 1-3	Protein Days
	Days 4-7	Weight Loss Menu Days
Week 2	Day 8	Protein Day
	Days 9-14	Weight Loss Menu Days
Week 3	Day 15	Protein Day
	Days 16-21	Weight Loss Menu Days
Week 4	Day 22	Protein Day
	Days 23-28	Weight Loss Menu Days

After completing a maximum of 28 days on Weight Loss, you'll then begin the Metabolic Adjustment portion of Phase 1. Completing Metabolic Adjustment after 28 days of Weight Loss is important *whether or not* you have reached your final goal weight.

METABOLIC ADJUSTMENT—14 DAYS

Day 1	Protein Day
Days 2-3	Metabolic Adjustment, Level 1
Days 4-7	Metabolic Adjustment, Level 2
Day 8	Protein Day
Days 9-14	Metabolic Adjustment, Level 3

Once you've successfully completed Metabolic Adjustment, you'll have a decision to make. If you want to lose more weight, you may begin another Weight Loss module of up to 28 days, followed by another Metabolic Adjustment period. If you've achieved your weight loss goal, you'll proceed directly from Metabolic Adjustment to "Phase 2: Lifetime Maintenance."

"PHASE 2: LIFETIME MAINTENANCE"

In the first three to six months of "Phase 2: Lifetime Maintenance" you'll gradually add a variety of foods to your diet. You'll learn how to achieve "metabolic equilibrium" and stabilize at your new lean weight so that you'll be able to appropriately eat a wider variety of foods and consume more calories without gaining weight.

EAT BETTER, MOVE MORE, STRESS LESS:
The Lean for Life Mantra for
Healthy Weight Management

As you do the Lean for Life program, you will learn how to:

"EAT BETTER"

Even if you can't always eat perfectly, you *can* "Eat Better." By increasing your awareness of what you're eating every day you can learn to make better food choices. We're here to help you learn how to fuel your body—and satisfy your taste buds—in ways that will support your weight loss goal.

"MOVE MORE"

You may not be able to exercise for a continuous hour every day (or even a half-hour every day), but you can "Move More"—more than you might have if you weren't so aware. During your program, you'll come to appreciate the benefits of moving more, and discover easy ways to build activity into your normal daily routine.

"STRESS LESS"

In response to chronic stress, you produce hormones that signal your body to store fat. This hormonal response to chronic stress speeds up the aging process, interferes with memory, damages vital organs and can cause premature death. It negatively affects us by interfering with our enjoyment of daily living. Stress is one of the major reasons people cite for abandoning a weight loss program. But no matter how hectic or demanding your life is, you can always "stress less," even if you can't be perfectly relaxed. During your program you will discover new ways to better manage the inevitable stress that life presents you.

A PERSONAL JOURNEY

Throughout every page of this book, my goal is to be your guide, to lead you on a journey that will be both enlightening and effective. During this process, I'll share stories of people who were once where you are now, wondering how to begin the program and what to expect.

At Lindora, we learned much of what we know from the experience and stories of real people. But there's one person's story that's especially close to my heart. If it weren't for her, it's unlikely this program would exist.

A few weeks after I started working on the first edition of this book, I was sitting at my dining room table, surrounded by reference material. Rather than sifting through the research, I found myself gazing out the window and thinking about my Grandma Angie, the woman whose battle with obesity inspired my father to develop what was to become Lindora Medical Clinics.

My grandmother was a bosomy, robust woman with a rich Southern drawl, a big laugh, and an even bigger heart. For as long as I can remember, she had always been a very large woman. Once, when I couldn't have been more than five or six years old, I was sitting on the

THE BENEFITS OF THE LEAN FOR LIFE PROGRAM

If you've ever tried traditional dieting—and who hasn't?—you know what an uphill struggle it can be. You think about food and are nagged by cravings. You often feel sluggish or irritable. If and when you do lose weight, it's typically a slow, tedious process.

On the *Lean for Life* program, you'll lose weight rapidly, burning excess body fat as fuel at the fastest rate possible, while maintaining your lean muscle mass. What's more, you'll have fewer cravings and feel less hungry. You'll experience increased energy and feel terrific!

LEAN FOR LIFE	TRADITIONAL DIETING
Rapid, safe weight loss	Slow weight loss
Reduced hunger	Increased hunger
Fewer cravings	More cravings
Increased energy	Decreased energy
Elevated mood	Often irritable
Maintain lean muscle mass	Lose muscle
Focus on lifestyle change	Focus on food plan

"It's never too late

to be who you

might have been."

— George Eliot

bed as she undressed. I had never seen her without a dress on and I remember being mesmerized by her mammoth thighs.

I was too young at the time to understand the health risks associated with carrying so many extra pounds, just as I was too young to know where the pounds came from in the first place.

Grandma Angie was a fabulous cook and I loved watching her prepare one of her specialties—large, soft pieces of fat fried in a heavy, blackened iron skillet. I can still taste the crisp, bacony pieces of fat and the squares of fried bread that she prepared in the leftover liquid fat.

Unfortunately, she didn't realize that the high fat, high calorie foods she lovingly prepared were contributing to a deadly disease process. One Christmas Eve, several years later, the holiday spirit was shattered when she nearly died of congestive heart failure. I remember feeling totally helpless as the ambulance pulled away, its shrill siren fading into the night. Not too long after that, my grandmother died from complications of obesity.

I know all too well the toll that excess weight can take. I'm the granddaughter of a wonderful woman who died too soon because she ate too much. I'm the daughter of a man whose passion for helping overweight people has had a major impact in shaping the way I think about diet, health, and fitness. I'm the mother of a nine-year-old daughter, determined to raise her with a healthy body—and a healthy body image—in a culture that reveres frightfully thin models as the feminine ideal. I'm also someone who lost weight on this program 30 years ago and who continues to practice its principles to maintain my weight today. I'm passionate about the Lean for Life program and am proud and delighted to be able to share it with you.

PREPARING FOR THE JOURNEY

While every person who chooses to do this program shares a common goal—to become Lean for Life—the path you travel is yours alone. In the coming weeks, you'll have many opportunities to look at the big picture as well as the details of your life. You'll clarify what works for you and what you'd like to change.

Together, we'll be doing important work. By the time you finish this book, you will have lost a significant amount of weight. You'll understand why conventional diets don't work and how you may well have contributed to your own frustration in your previous efforts to lose weight. You'll also become knowledgeable about the ways in which your body gains and loses fat, and how you can tip the scale in your favor. You'll discover what works and, just as important, what doesn't.

You're about to set out on an empowering journey of weight loss, self-improvement, and self-discovery that will result in your looking better, feeling healthier, and being more fully equipped than ever to meet whatever challenges life offers you.

For some, this process represents an exciting new beginning, a fresh start. They will experience a renewed sense of focus and a stronger commitment to themselves. They will see it as a great adventure and will be eager to seize the day.

For others, the process brings with it an element of apprehension. Having lost weight in the past, only to regain it, they're more likely to be cautiously optimistic. They believe in the program, sometimes more than they believe in themselves, and are willing to "try it," but they won't be entirely convinced it will "work" for them until they do it.

How are you feeling right now? Are you enthusiastic? Ambivalent? Afraid? Whatever emotions you're experiencing, what ultimately matters isn't what you're *feeling* but what you're *doing*. You've chosen to make something positive happen for yourself, and you've already taken some major steps.

Your journey to becoming Lean for Life will be different, because you will decide how far you want to go and how quickly you want to get there. You will learn how to get back on the path if you happen to lose your way.

Along the way, remember three things:

1. You're making this journey *for* yourself, but not *by* yourself. This book will be your companion and supporter along the way, as will the men and women who will share their stories with you within its pages. You'll also have access to a support system that can include our clinical staff, our website (www.leanforlife.com), and one-on-one telephone coaching.

2. You will accomplish your goal of better health and a better body, but not by doing the same things you've done in the past. You will learn to travel lighter, leaving behind the baggage of past dieting experiences and picking up new tools, strategies, and techniques.

3. You have the time you need to accomplish all you want. You're beginning a lifelong journey where quick fixes don't exist. Establishing new habits takes time. Please know that you can maintain your own pace as you work for lasting change.

This book is designed to guide you, day-by-day, through the program, introducing new ideas and information along the way. What you learn tomorrow will build upon what you learn today. At Lindora, we know from clinical experience that most people find it much easier to learn and apply new information when they are exposed to it gradually. We call this learning process the "drip method." So rather than being flooded with chapters of concepts and theory before you have an understanding of how to apply any of it, I urge you to follow step-by-step and apply to your own life what's presented each day. Soon, you'll discover for yourself the issues that contributed to your weight gain and the solutions for lasting change.

If you fall behind on your reading on any given day, don't panic or get discouraged. Simply make a note to read those pages the following day. It's also a good idea to review the material from earlier days as you continue through the program. People often comment that they're amazed at how much good information they missed the first time through, or how the information takes on a new relevance each time they read it.

A Lean for Life Success Story

DIANA ROSENFELD

"I was never an unattractive woman—just well hidden. I've lost more than 400 pounds on the Lean for Life program. In the process, I've gained a degree of self-esteem and self-respect that is helping me redefine my life."

THEN & NOW

CREATING YOUR OWN SUCCESS STORY

This book is a collaborative effort in the truest sense of the word. It's not only a collaboration among the thousands of Lindora clients and "Team Lindora" employees whose collective wisdom and personal experience it reflects, but ultimately it's a collaboration between us. You. And me. That's because *Lean for Life* is not simply a book you read. It's a book you do. And until you make it come to life by doing the program it provides, it's merely words on a page.

The most important story has yet to be written. It's yours. Unlike a novel, in which the author's imagination determines the fate of the main character, how this book ends is ultimately up to you. It's *your* success story—one *you* are about to create.

If you're ready, let's get started.

FACING THE FEAR

Fear of failure. It's the single most common reason for not starting a weight loss program. If you've ever dieted and not lost weight—or regained whatever weight you did lose—some degree of apprehension is natural.

The question is how to deal with that fear. Will you manage it or will it manage you? It's easy to let fear surface in the form of excuses: "I'm too stressed and busy to start anything new right now," "I always gain it back anyway, so what's the point?," "I don't really feel that bad." But will statements like these help you achieve your weight loss goal?

The Lean for Life program is probably different from diets you've tried in the past. Lean for Life offers a rare opportunity for you to learn and practice life-management skills while losing weight. Take the time to read several of the "Lean for Life Success Stories" featured throughout the book. You can be sure every one of these people experienced episodes of fear and self-doubt along the way. And yet they did it. They were determined to overcome the fear of failure in order to earn the pride of accomplishment. They succeeded. You can, too.

'THE SIX ESSENTIALS' FOR SUCCESS

What is the difference between those who *succeed* on the Lean for Life program and those who simply try? Those who succeed have learned to integrate Dr. Stamper's "Six Essentials" into their daily lives.

The "Six Essentials" are powerful, fundamental truths that will guide you in achieving the weight loss results you want. They have been developed and refined over more than 30 years at our 31 Southern California clinics. They are such a cornerstone of the Lean for Life program that you will find one or more of them addressed, in one way or another, on virtually every page of this book. In fact, some of our most successful clients make a game of identifying which of "The Six Essentials" are featured in each day's chapter.

"I call them the Six Essentials," Dr. Stamper explains, "because I'm convinced that once you understand these concepts and master them, you'll never again need to diet. You will truly *be* Lean for Life."

The human body is amazingly complex. The "Six Essentials" distill the experience we've gained through more than ten million patient visits at Lindora Medical Clinics. They are a simple way of explaining complicated mind-body processes in a way that can be quickly understood so you can then apply solutions that we have found to be effective.

THE SIX ESSENTIALS

1. Make your goal "to **learn** to be lean for life."

2. Your level of **interest and enthusiasm** will determine your level of success.

3. Learn to recognize and **eliminate your defensive barriers.**

4. Learn to **control cravings.**

5. Learn to **use relaxation techniques** and "stress less."

6. **Follow the maintenance program** for lasting success.

ESSENTIAL #1: MAKE YOUR GOAL "TO LEARN TO BE LEAN FOR LIFE"

Everything we do successfully begins with a goal. Unfortunately, most people who want to lose weight tend to focus on a number—"I want to lose 35 pounds"—rather than on the type of goal that will help them achieve lasting success.

Dr. Stamper tells clients: "The human brain is a goal-seeking organism, so it's vital that you establish the *appropriate* goals to achieve your desired results." Diets don't work for the long term because they tend to focus on a temporary change in dietary composition. With Lean for Life, the focus is on *learning* to become lean. The process of learning creates new neural connections within your brain. These new connections create actual structural changes in your brain. With reinforcement (practice), the changes (connections) can become permanent, and before long, you'll find that making healthy choices about what you eat seems like second nature. And it will be! Your process for decision making will have been permanently changed. To achieve true weight control, form those new neural connections and make your primary goal to *learn* to become lean for *life.*

Those who commit to this learning process are the ones who ultimately achieve lifetime weight control. "The learning aspect of the goal is the challenging part," says Dr. Stamper. "However, it is learning about problems and their solutions that leads to becoming Lean for Life."

ESSENTIAL #2: YOUR LEVEL OF INTEREST AND ENTHUSIASM WILL DETERMINE YOUR LEVEL OF SUCCESS

The greater your interest and enthusiasm for achieving your goal, the more likely you are to achieve it.

Achieving any goal requires an investment of energy, and that energy is sustained when you're motivated to continue striving to reach your goal. The problem, of course, is that motivation wavers. In fact, for some dieters, it often only lasts until the next meal! That's why on page 49, we encourage you to create your personal "Motivator Cards", a list of all the benefits you'll enjoy when you become Lean for Life. By posting your cards on your bathroom mirror, in your car, and at work where you'll see them every day, you're much more likely to maintain interest and enthusiasm in your goal because you'll be reminded of why you started the program in the first place.

Motivation without adequate information, however, leads to frustration. That's why it's also important for you to read this book every day during your program. Make a daily commitment to review these "Six Essentials" and incorporate them into your life. Your level of interest and enthusiasm *will* determine your level of success.

ESSENTIAL #3: LEARN TO RECOGNIZE AND ELIMINATE YOUR DEFENSIVE BARRIERS

We all have defensive barriers that we unconsciously use to protect ourselves from painful realities. It's essential to learn to recognize and eliminate our personal defensive barriers because when they're operating, we're not fully open to growth and change. Defensive barriers sabotage our goals and impair our ability to learn.

The two commonly used defensive barriers that have a great impact on weight management are *denial* and *rationalization*. Denial, which we'll discuss in depth on "Day 6: The Denial Trap" (pages 95-102), is an unwillingness or refusal to accept or admit a reality. Rationalization, which we'll explore on "Day 7: Recognizing Rationalization" (pages 103-108), is an excuse our minds make up to help us feel better about an undesirable or inappropriate behavior or situation.

Have you ever caught yourself saying "Oh, one little bite won't kill me!" or "I deserve this—I've been good all day!" And how about this one: "I don't need to write down what I eat—I have a great memory!" Accepting that we all use denial and rationalization can be difficult, but acknowledging that we do is a fundamental, giant step toward lasting success. You can learn to recognize and eliminate defensive barriers by applying the success strategies featured on pages 104-105. This will help ward off excuses and denial.

ESSENTIAL #4: LEARN TO CONTROL CRAVINGS

Dieters don't fail to achieve their lean weight goal because they lack willpower. They fail because of cravings. "Cravings" are those urges to eat that you experience even when you're not hungry. Although this urge to eat may often seem to appear out of nowhere, cravings are actually the result of various physical, psychological, and environmental factors that affect the way your brain and your body function. A word of warning from Dr. Stamper: "All three causes must be dealt with, because a craving is dangerous to your program."

Once you understand the causes of cravings and learn the solutions for overcoming them, you'll be on your way to being lean for *life!*"

DR. STAMPER

"All three causes of cravings must be dealt with, because a craving is dangerous to your program."

I. Physical Causes of Cravings

The overweight body is different from that of a naturally lean person's body in regard to certain functions that affect appetite and fat storage. There are four basic differences:

1.   Elevated Setpoint

The human body is designed to store fat and then burn it as fuel. It strives to maintain body weight (fat stores) within a relatively narrow range to ensure that there is an adequate amount of fuel available when needed. A part of the brain called the hypothalamus works to accomplish this weight "stability" by regulating the appetite and metabolism—the rate at which calories are burned. We refer to this control mechanism as the appestat or "setpoint".

The setpoint can be elevated by prolonged periods of overeating, pregnancy, surgery, or anything else that affects food intake and activity over a period of time. Once the setpoint becomes elevated, the body strives to maintain a higher weight and will increase the appetite and lower the metabolism to accomplish this goal. Because of this, the overweight person's appetite and hunger is more severe than a naturally lean person who does not have an elevated setpoint.

This situation is compounded when the overweight person tries to lose weight by simply eating less. Their elevated setpoint attempts to cause their body to maintain its current weight by increasing hunger and cravings, making it very uncomfortable for the dieter to eat less. They feel sluggish, irritable, and often experience mood swings. In addition, the dieter's rate of weight loss can be extremely slow as their metabolism lowers in response to the decreased food intake.

The Solution: A ketogenic weight loss program provides many benefits that can help "bypass" the setpoint and make the weight loss experience more comfortable and effective. In addition to a rapid rate of weight loss, most people who are in a state of dietary ketosis experience a decrease in hunger and cravings. They generally don't experience the irritability and mood swings that often accompany traditional dieting. Pages 19-21 provide a more detailed description of dietary ketosis, how it works, and how it benefits you while you're on the Lean for Life program.

2. Insulin Resistance

Our body converts the food we eat to glucose. Insulin helps glucose pass through the membranes of the muscle cells so it can be used for fuel. Being overweight and inactive can impair the body's ability to utilize insulin, making it difficult for insulin to get the glucose into the cells. The impairment of your body's ability to use insulin is referred to as "insulin resistance." As insulin resistance builds, the body tries to compensate by producing more insulin. This becomes a vicious cycle, however, because the presence of insulin also signals the body to store more fat, which then creates even more resistance. In addition, glucose and insulin levels fluctuate, causing hunger and cravings to overeat. As this cycle continues, it can lead to serious health conditions such as diabetes, high blood pressure, elevated cholesterol, and cardiovascular disease.

The Solution: When you correctly follow the Lean for Life program, your glucose and insulin levels can stabilize very quickly and your hunger will be reduced. Current research indicates the problem of insulin resistance not only can be slowed but can actually be reversed by weight loss and regular physical activity.

3. Inadequate Mitochondrial Surface

Mitochondria are tiny, egg-shaped structures in your cells that act as fat-burning furnaces. To explain a complex process simply, they receive the nutrients from the blood stream and burn them for energy. The more mitrochrondial surface you have in your cells, the easier it is for your body to burn fat for fuel. Overweight people don't have enough mitochondria to burn all that they have eaten, and the remainder is stored as fat. As more fat is stored, insulin resistance increases and the setpoint elevates, which creates a cycle of increased hunger and cravings, increased food intake and fat storage.

The Solution: Increase physical activity. Moderate exercise develops more mitochondrial surface in the muscles and increases your ability to burn fat for fuel. In addition, exercise improves your body's ability to move glucose from the blood stream into the cells. This helps stabilize glucose and insulin levels, which in turn decreases hunger and cravings. So as you see, the benefits of exercise extend far beyond simply burning calories!

All you need to do is forty-five minutes of moderate exercise per day, five days a week. And you don't even have to do it all at once.

Fifteen minutes, three times a day, will make a difference! What constitutes "moderate exercise"? We discuss it in depth on "Day 3: Moderate Exercise and Magical Mitochrondria" (pages 73-79).

4. Low or Fluctuating Serotonin Levels

Serotonin is a powerful neurotransmitter that regulates mood, hunger, and eating behavior. When serotonin levels are low, one may experience excessive hunger, frequent carbohydrate cravings, and feel irritable, moody, or depressed. For some people, being overweight is directly related to low serotonin levels.

Although many people find that a state of dietary ketosis adequately controls hunger and cravings during weight loss, those with low serotonin levels may need additional help to achieve control.

The Solution: Studies suggest that aerobic exercise such as jogging and dancing boost serotonin levels. Safe, effective medications that regulate serotonin levels are also currently available by prescription. Although such medications may not be appropriate for everyone, those who need it often experience excellent results when taking them. Consult with your physician if you think you might benefit from such medications.

II. Psychological Causes of Cravings: The Self-Image of Fatness

The brain operates on two levels—the conscious and the subconscious. When you operate on a conscious level, you're aware, thinking, and evaluating that which you see and hear. The subconscious level, however, is like a computer that functions automatically, responding to information and perceptions that have been "programmed" into it over a period of time.

The self-image is a function of the subconscious level. From the moment we're born, we receive messages from our environment and the people around us about who we are and how our lives are supposed to be. Whether or not these messages are true, our subconscious brain absorbs them and incorporates them into our belief system. Once our self-image has been formed in our "computer," we cannot easily vary from it. Our behavior, thoughts, and reactions are rooted in our self-image.

When your subconscious self-image is one of an overweight person, you may sometimes feel as if you're two different people. One part of you wants to follow your weight control program, while the other part sabotages your efforts. When faced with a challenging situation, it's your self-image that determines your response. For example, if you're facing temptation and are thinking, "I'll never be able to eat well during the holidays!", that's your fat self-image at work.

The Solution: Reprogram your self-image from "overweight" to "lean." Until you accomplish this, you will experience a subconscious pressure to remain overweight. So how do you reprogram your own self image? By practicing thought control, positive affirmations, and mental imagery every day. The S.T.O.P. model on page 86 is a valuable tool to use when cravings occur. Explanations and examples of these powerful tools can be found throughout this book. You'll find "Day 18: Your Mental Blueprint: Who—and How—are You Supposed to Be?" (pages 165-168) especially valuable.

III. Environmental Causes of Cravings: The Conditioned Eating Response

Over time, we develop the habit of eating in response to certain "triggers" in our lives. These triggers may be related to specific events, places, emotions, or people. For example, if you eat every time you get bored or angry, it eventually becomes a habit and you'll continually turn to food whenever you experience these emotions. Many people have developed the habit of eating popcorn whenever they go to the movies. Every time they walk into a movie theatre, or even think about going to see a movie, they crave popcorn. Some people even have "eating buddies"—they eat every time they get together. Over time, this becomes a habit and they experience the urge to eat whether or not their plans include a meal.

When you have a conditioned eating response, you react without thinking. You may experience the urge to eat even without being aware of what triggered the craving.

The Solution: Become aware of your eating triggers and change your response by using a process for changing behavior that we refer to as **D.D.P.P.**:

Desire: Nothing happens until we truly want it to. Psych yourself up every day. Develop motivational habits.

Decision: "Wanting" is not enough. You must decide to make it happen. Your decision to stay committed and follow the Lean for Life program is one you'll make many times every day.

Plan of Action: You need a specific, detailed plan for how you will guide your behavior into successful patterns. A Plan of Action allows you to maintain greater control when facing the inevitable day-to-day challenges that can trigger cravings. Think of your Plan of Action as a road map. Use it and it will help guide you to your destination.

Perseverance: Make a commitment to stay focused—to "stick with it"— until you accomplish your goal. As an old Broadway song suggests, "It's not where you start, it's where you finish!"

You'll discover other proven, practical solutions to overcoming the environmental causes of cravings on "Day 5: Cravings Caused By People, Places, Emotions and Events" (pages 88-94).

ESSENTIAL #5: LEARN TO USE RELAXATION TECHNIQUES AND STRESS LESS

Time and time again, researchers see the same pattern emerge: people who have difficulty managing stress also have difficulty losing weight. And when they manage to lose weight, they usually regain it. Instead of learning to identify and manage stress in healthy ways, many people turn to food as a coping mechanism. To compound the problem, chronic stress causes the body to release a hormone called cortisol, which stimulates the body to increase fat stores. What's more, other stress hormones can even kill neurons in our brains (that's a scary thought!), making it harder to think clearly when we need to most!

The Solution: In order to stop using food as a "tranquilizer", it's essential that you learn other techniques for managing stress. There are a number of healthy alternatives to "stress eating," including regular physical activity, meditation, listening to relaxation tapes, and deep breathing exercises. On "Day 11: Learn to Manage Stress and You'll Learn to Manage Food" (pages 124-130), you'll discover an effective technique for rubbing out your neck muscles that will literally allow you to take stress management into your own hands!

We may not be able to completely eliminate stressful situations from our lives, but we can choose healthy ways to deal with them. Learning to manage stress—instead of allowing it to manage you—is an essential step to becoming Lean for Life.

ESSENTIAL #6: FOLLOW THE MAINTENANCE PROGRAM FOR LASTING SUCCESS

How long do you plan to maintain your new, lean weight? Do you want to be lean for life or just lean for a while? Did you know that a large percentage of the people who lose weight gain it back within one to five years—and that they could have *prevented* that regain by following a comprehensive maintenance plan?

Spending time and money to lose weight and then not following through with a program that will help you maintain your new lean weight isn't a very productive choice. It's like going to your doctor with a broken leg, spending money for x-rays and a cast, and then deciding on your own to remove the cast early. You wouldn't consider doing such a thing, would you? You wouldn't because you know there would be negative consequences, namely that your leg wouldn't heal properly.

When you get a haircut, do you ever assume it will be your last? You don't, because you know that no matter how terrific your hair may look when you get it cut, it requires maintenance to stay looking the way you want it. Your body is no different. Once you lose the weight, a maintenance program is essential in order to maintain the benefits.

A "maintenance" program or system involves more than just knowing what to eat. It provides focus and structure (like a cast for a broken leg) as you actively incorporate specific success strategies and principles into your daily life.

It's essential to understand that a period of long-term weight maintenance is required to allow your setpoint to adjust to a normal level in order to prevent weight regain. If this isn't done, you'll be unable to eat "normally" without regaining. As Dr. Stamper explains: "As long as your setpoint remains elevated, it will divert calories normally used for energy and repair of the body into stored fat until all of your lost weight is regained." Pages 241-242 provide more information about the three- to twelve-month process of adjusting the setpoint.

WARNING: Not following a weight maintenance plan once you've achieved your goal weight is detrimental to your long-term success. Do you remember the quote from Anne Kaiser Stearns on the first page of this book? It reads, "If you always do what you've always done, you'll always get what you always got." When it comes to maintenance, consider this: "If you want something different, you've got to *do* something different."

PHASE 1: WEIGHT LOSS

During the Weight Loss module of the Lean for Life program, you'll be following a low calorie, low carbohydrate, low fat, moderate protein structured eating plan designed to help you achieve safe, rapid weight loss. Whenever you significantly limit your intake of carbohydrates—your body's primary energy source—and total calories for a long enough period of time, you'll reach a point where your body draws on its alternate energy system, fat stores, for fuel. This means your body burns fat and turns it into a source of fuel called ketones. In other words, you recycle your stored body fat. Body fat, which was once food, becomes fuel again.

When you burn a larger amount of fat than is immediately needed for energy, the excess ketones are eliminated in the urine. Throughout the Weight Loss module, you'll know you're burning excess fat because you'll be monitoring your urine with a ketone-measuring strip, or "ketostick," every morning. Ketone sticks measure the amount of ketones in the urine. At Lindora, we refer to these ketone sticks as the "FBI"—Fat Burning Indicators.™ The reactive pad on the end of the ketone stick changes color when a significant amount of ketones come into contact with it. If your ketone stick registers a positive reading—a range from pink to purple color—you're "in ketosis." If it doesn't change color, you'll know you've consumed too many carbohydrates during a recent meal or snack and are primarily using carbohydrates for fuel instead of burning excess fat.

"We must begin where we are, wherever that is. Small steps will lead to larger steps."

— Peg Thompson

Many people tell us they like using the ketone sticks because they provide objective and reliable confirmation that the program is working. If you already have your ketosticks, you might want to test your urine now. Since you haven't started the Weight Loss plan, it's unlikely that you'll "show color" yet, but at least you'll have a point of reference. You'll know what a negative result looks like. You'll also reinforce the fact that when you're not following the plan, your ketostick will be negative.

THE BENEFITS OF DIETARY KETOSIS

An eating plan that results in dietary ketosis is called a "ketogenic diet." Since Lindora was founded back in 1971, thousands of weight loss programs have been introduced through books, magazine articles, television shows, infomercials, and advertising. So why, with so many options and approaches available, has Lindora used a ketogenic weight loss program for more than thirty years? Because of the many benefits— and excellent results—that hundreds of thousands of people have experienced on the Lean for Life program while in dietary ketosis.

People who diligently follow the Lean for Life program experience safe, rapid weight loss. Because they tend to lose weight more quickly than on traditional diets that focus strictly on calories, their motivation to stick with the program until they achieve their goal is great. They also experience reduced hunger and fewer cravings. People in dietary ketosis also report experiencing increased physical and mental energy. They consistently tell us they feel less moody, less irritable, and less depressed. Patients in our clinic program often report feeling euphoric while in ketosis. The degree to which people experience these benefits varies from person to person, but you can reasonably expect to feel better as you progress on your Lean for Life program.

A Lindora study headed by clinical psychologist Harry K. Wexler, Ph.D., published in August, 2001, showed that participation in our medically supervised weight loss program resulted not only in weight loss, but in significant improvements in a broad range of psychological variables during six weeks of weight loss by participants who were mildly to severely depressed at the beginning of the study.

Upon admission to the study, 317 overweight female volunteers completed a packet of self-report questionnaires. One hundred sixty of the volunteers, or 54% of the initial group, were found to be mildly to severely depressed. Of this group, 43.7% were mildly depressed, 37.5% were moderately depressed, and 18.8% were severely depressed.

The volunteers were assessed again after their third and sixth weeks on the Lindora program. Their scores indicating depression significantly decreased at three weeks, and by the end of the sixth week on the program, all psychological variables were found to be within the normal range.

IS KETOSIS SAFE?

Dietary ketosis is one of the most maligned and misunderstood concepts in the world of health and nutrition. It is often confused with ketoacidosis, which is a life-threatening condition associated with uncontrolled insulin-deficient Type 1 diabetes. Ketoacidosis occurs in the Type 1 diabetic when the absence of insulin leads to a toxic build-up of blood glucose and an extreme breakdown of fat and muscle tissue. This condition does not occur in individuals who have even a small amount of insulin, whether from natural production or artifically administered.

Dietary ketosis, on the other hand, is a natural adjustment to the body's reduced intake of carbohydrates as it shifts its primary source of energy from carbohydrates to excess stored fat. The presence of insulin keeps ketone production in check so that a mild, beneficial ketosis is achieved. Blood glucose levels are stabilized within a normal range and there is no breakdown of healthy muscle tissue.

The most sensitive tests of ketosis ("NMR" and "blood ketone level") show that virtually everyone is in some degree of ketosis every day, particularly in the early morning after having not eaten over a period of hours. Ketosis is a normal metabolic process to help the body meet its energy needs during periods of reduced food intake. Ketosis is the body's survival system. The body functions naturally and effectively while in a state of dietary ketosis. It is not an abnormality, nor does it present any medical danger, except to a Type 1 insulin-dependent diabetic.

A MOTIVATING RATE OF WEIGHT LOSS

The rate of weight loss experienced on the Lean for Life program is safe and motivating. Our clients lose an average of two to five pounds per week during the Weight Loss module. The amount you lose can be influenced by individual variables such as age, gender, starting weight, level of physical activity, and how strictly you follow the program. If you don't lose all the weight you want to lose during your first cycle through Phase 1, you may repeat the process as needed until you achieve your Lean for Life goal. Repeating the process means doing up to four more weeks of Weight Loss, followed by another two weeks of Metabolic Adjustment. You can repeat this six-week process until you reach your lean weight, at which point you will begin "Phase 2: Lifetime Maintenance."

If you are following this program under clinical supervision, your clinician may recommend Weight Loss modules of up to eight weeks, followed by two weeks of Metabolic Adjustment. The individual monitoring and professional guidance that you receive from trained clinicians allows for greater program flexibility.

CAN ANYONE DO A KETOGENIC PROGRAM?

While ketosis is a normal part of the body's fat-burning process, there are some people for whom a ketogenic weight loss program is NOT recommended:

- **Women who are pregnant or nursing.** Expectant mothers should not follow a ketogenic weight loss program. We also recommend that nursing mothers wait until they finish breastfeeding before starting the Lean for Life program, as it's unclear whether a nursing mother being in mild dietary ketosis could affect the baby. In addition, being on a weight loss diet with decreased calorie intake and food restrictions can decrease breast milk production and may otherwise have a negative effect on the baby's optimal health and well-being.

- **People with serious liver or kidney disease.** People with kidney or liver disease may have specific dietary or other restrictions that are not compatible with a ketogenic program. Consult your physician regarding whether this program is appropriate for you.

- **Type 1, insulin-dependent diabetics.** A Type 1 diabetic's food intake and insulin regime must be *very strictly* monitored and carefully balanced to prevent them from going into a state of ketoacidosis.

If you have any concerns or questions, be sure to consult with your health care professional before beginning this program.

HOW WILL I FEEL WHILE ON THE PROGRAM?

It's a question that's asked every day in our clinics and on our website. The answer varies as much as the people who ask it. Many people feel terrific from the very first day. They marvel at the fact that they're not hungry, and comment on their increased energy and overall sense of well-being.

Others, however, find the process more challenging, occasionally experiencing *temporary food withdrawal symptoms* such as headache, fatigue, irritability, insomnia, fluid retention, nausea and/or indigestion.

If this happens to you, don't be alarmed. It's perfectly normal for your body to react whenever you make significant changes in the way you eat. I tell you this not because you *will* experience any symptoms or side effects, but because it's possible that you *may.*

One of the best passages I've seen on food withdrawal symptoms comes from a book called *Forever Thin* by Theodore Isaac Rubin, M.D. In discussing food addiction, Dr. Rubin explains that when a person's "normal" food supply is in any way curtailed, the individual may experience both physical and psychological reactions that can vary in degree and are sometimes mistaken for other illness. Writes Rubin: "There may be digestive, respiratory, urinary, circulatory, and emotional disturbances in any number of combinations. There may be constipation, diarrhea, heartburn, indigestion, gas pains, spasms, cramps, air swallowing, urinary retention, urinary frequency, irregular heartbeat, rapid heartbeat, chest pain, shortness of breath, itching, etc., etc., etc., as well as depression, anxiety, irritability, fatigue, insomnia, excessive smoking, agitation, excessive worry, nightmares, unusual fears, etc., etc."

You may take over-the-counter remedies to relieve symptoms, such as aspirin, acetaminophen or ibuprofen for headache, and antacid tablets for heartburn or indigestion. Correctly following the program guidelines on pages 29-31 can help eliminate or reduce the severity of any food withdrawal symptoms you may experience.

As discussed later in this chapter, one of the consequences of reducing carbohydrate intake is a reduction in body fluid. This can result in a lowering of blood pressure. For people who normally have high blood pressure, this is an added benefit. In fact, if you are taking medication for high blood pressure, talk with your doctor. You may find, over time, it's necessary to reduce your dosage.

If your blood pressure tends to be normal or lower than normal, it's possible that, because of a reduction in body fluid and the resulting lower blood pressure, you may experience light-headedness and dizziness, especially when standing up quickly. If this happens, don't panic. Stand up more slowly and allow your body to adjust. **To maintain adequate blood pressure, make sure you're getting enough salt in your diet.** You may want to monitor your blood pressure during Weight Loss if you experience these symptoms.

Please review the information about potassium and sodium supplementation on pages 25-26 regarding symptoms of fatigue, muscle weakness and/or cramps.

Overall, you should expect to feel energetic and healthy when you follow the program correctly.

VITAMIN AND MINERAL SUPPLEMENTS

Vitamins are an essential part of the Lean for Life program. They help maximize absorption and utilization of the food you eat, as well as safeguard against nutritional deficiencies. Weight loss can increase the body's need for vitamins and minerals above the United States Recommended Daily Allowance (USRDA). The USRDA for vitamins and minerals represents the lowest levels at which the body is able to ward off disease, but not necessarily the level for optimal performance. The Lean for Life vitamin and mineral supplement has been developed to augment our weight loss program.

Our clinical experience has shown that those who use these vitamins and minerals feel better while on the program.

The Lean for Life vitamin with mineral supplement is available in our Lindora clinics and may also be ordered by mail or phone. Please see the Resources section of this book for more information. If you're not doing the program under clinical supervision and choose not to use the Lean for Life vitamin supplements, be sure that you select a high-quality multi-vitamin and mineral supplement that exceeds the USRDA.

ESSENTIAL FATTY ACIDS

Essential fatty acids serve important metabolic roles in providing the necessary building blocks for the body's normal growth, repair, and normal function. Two fatty acids, linoleic and alpha linoleic acid, cannot be produced by the body and therefore must be supplied in the diet. Use two tablespoons (one ounce) of safflower, flaxseed, soybean, or corn oil *per week*, or essential fatty acid capsules taken as directed, to prevent deficiency. See page 35 for more information.

CALCIUM

People who are on a weight loss program may occasionally require additional calcium supplementation. It is usually recommended that pre-menopausal women take about 1,000-1,200 mg. of calcium per day and post-menopausal take 1,500 mg. of calcium per day. This level of supplementation will usually be sufficient to prevent any symptom of low calcium and will help guard against osteoporosis. However, should symptoms of a "pins and needles" sensation occur around the mouth or in the fingers, additional calcium may be required.

POTASSIUM AND SODIUM

Potassium is a mineral that is necessary for all living cells. It helps to maintain proper electrolyte balance in body cells, is essential for proper muscle function, and is instrumental in conducting nerve impulses.

While most people get the potassium they need—50 to 100 milliequivalents (meq.) per day—from the foods they eat, there are occasions when one may need extra potassium. The body's potassium reserves can become depleted, for example, when there is an excessive loss of fluid through diarrhea, vomiting, or the use of some diuretics and laxatives. Similarly, the body can lose potassium any time there is a large flow of urine, as may happen when carbohydrate intake is restricted and when a person is drinking a lot of fluids.

If your blood potassium level is low, it's wise to take enough potassium to raise and maintain it in the mid-normal to high-normal range. Muscle weakness and/or muscle cramps are symptoms strongly suggestive of a potassium deficiency, and merit prompt attention to prevent further depletion and such potentially serious consequences as irregularities in heart rhythm.

A day's supply of the Lean for Life vitamin and mineral supplement contains potassium, as do some of the Lean for Life protein products. The amount may not be adequate for everyone, however, so additional supplementation may be required. Lindora clinic patients take a prescription-strength potassium supplement during Phase 1 to maintain normal potassium levels—potassium chloride 750 mg. (10 mEq.). Potassium is also available over the counter in lower doses. Many people who do the Lean for Life program on their own (without medical supervision) tell us they take an over the counter potassium gluconate supplement during Phase 1 to prevent deficiency and the resulting symptoms. Most report they feel best when taking a 99 mg. tablet three times a day with meals. Participants who are especially active tend to take more than three tablets a day, as needed. Table salt and salt substitutes also contain potassium.

If you are being treated for a chronic disease, high blood pressure, or are taking potassium-sparing diuretics, you should not take extra potassium supplements without first consulting your physician or health-care professional.

Like potassium, sodium helps regulate the body's fluid balance. Sodium is present in the foods we eat, usually in adequate amounts to meet ordinary demands. Sodium levels may become depleted, however, when excessive body fluid is lost during times of profuse sweating, diarrhea and vomiting.

Normal sodium intake is usually enough to maintain an adequate amount of fluid in our blood vessels, and thus to maintain a normal blood pressure. The total amount of fluid within the blood vessels decreases, however, when people are on a low-carbohydrate weight loss program. As a result, blood pressure can drop, especially when a person stands suddenly from a seated or horizontal position, causing weakness, lightheadedness, and dizziness. This is called orthostatic hypotension (low blood pressure resulting from a change in position).

To prevent this, we encourage our patients who have low or normal blood pressure to add regular table salt to their food and/or drink one cup of boullion twice a day during the Weight Loss module. The resulting restoration of normal blood volume sometimes results in a temporary "water weight" increase, but any such gain is soon reversed as weight loss proceeds.

It's prudent to monitor your blood pressure during the program, especially if you experience any of the symptoms described. Low sodium levels can cause symptoms that are similar to potassium deficiency: dizziness, fatigue, lack of energy, muscle weakness and/or muscle cramps. If you experience these symptoms, particularly if you are already taking potassium, we encourage you to add extra table salt to your daily diet or drink a cup of prepared boullion twice a day. Table salt has the added benefit of containing potassium.

Your need for potassium and/or sodium supplementation may best be determined by consulting your physician or health-care professional. This is essential if you are taking medication regularly or being treated for a chronic disease. Your health care professional can obtain additional information about this and all other aspects of the Lean for Life program by calling 1-800-LINDORA.

Another Lean for Life Success Story

CLOVER BEHREND

At age 49, Clover Behrend was diagnosed with Type 2 diabetes. Four years later, in 1994, her condition was so out of control that she had to take insulin injections twice a day. In May, 2001, with the consent of her physician, Clover began the Lean for Life program.

"My diabetes was out of control," Clover recalls. "I was eating what I wanted, when I wanted, and I wasn't doing any physical activity. It was taking a toll on my body—and my spirit."

After losing 29 pounds on the Lean for Life program in just nine weeks, Clover says she's healthier than she has been in forty years.

"During the entire nine weeks on the Weight Loss phase of the Lean for Life program, I only needed two five-unit insulin injections, compared to two 15-unit injections a day before I started," Clover says. "I'm definitely liking the changes in my appearance, but what matters more to me is how I feel. I'm not sluggish or lethargic anymore. I'm eating so much better—who knew I could actually enjoy fruit more than a brownie? I'm sleeping more soundly and I'm moving more often—and more easily—than I have in a very long time. And best of all, my blood sugar is consistently within the range of a non-diabetic person!"

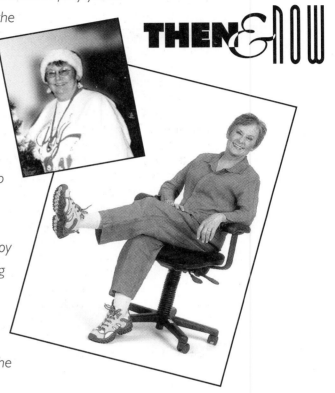

THEN&NOW

WEIGHT LOSS: STEP BY STEP

You will refer to these guidelines daily throughout Weight Loss.

You will begin the Weight Loss module of the program by following the *Prep Day* guidelines on pages 46-48. Once you've completed your Prep Days, you will do up to three *Initial Protein Days* as outlined on pages 29-33. After completing your Initial Protein Days, you will begin the *Weight Loss Menu Plan*, doing one Protein Day each week. Pages 33-39 feature the guidelines, Menu Plan, and Food Selection list. See pages 40-41 for Weekly Protein Day guidelines.

If your ketostick is negative at any time during the Weight Loss module, or you experience difficulty losing weight, you'll want to refer to pages 41-45. The information on these pages will help you evaluate your program and provides specific guidelines for a plan of action that will help you successfully move forward toward your lean weight goal.

INITIAL PROTEIN DAYS 1-3

After completing the three-day Prep, you will begin the Weight Loss module by doing a maximum of three Protein Days. The Protein Days will "jump start" your weight loss program and help you achieve the beneficial state of dietary ketosis. During your Protein Days, you'll be eating approximately 100 grams of protein a day, while keeping your carbohydrate intake low—somewhere in the neighborhood of 50-100 grams. This ensures that you will begin burning fat as rapidly as possible.

What distinguishes the Protein Days from the rest of the Weight Loss module is that you will be eating only protein-based foods—no fruits, vegetables, or other foods during this time. You will choose low carbohydrate, low fat, protein foods such as eggs or egg whites, tuna, turkey or chicken breast, low-fat tofu, and other foods from the Protein list on page 37. In addition, throughout the program—and especially during the Protein Days—many Lindora patients enjoy the convenience and variety of eating delicious, high-quality Lean for Life high protein nutritional products. (See pages 32-33 for more information.) By mixing and matching your protein food choices and Lean for Life protein products, you can enjoy a wide variety of tastes during your Protein Days.

HOW TO DO YOUR PROTEIN DAYS

❏ To achieve the fat-burning state of dietary ketosis, you will keep your carbohydrate intake somewhere in the range of approximately 50 to 100 grams a day. The exact number depends on the individual, so you'll need to experiment to determine the number that allows you to achieve and maintain ketosis. You'll know you're in ketosis if your ketostick shows a pink to purple color when you test your urine. It may take a few days for you to see good color on your ketostick. Lindora clinic patients usually start by having between 80 to 100 grams of carbohydrate on their first and second Protein Days. If not in ketosis by the morning of the third day, they decrease their carb intake to 70 to 80 grams, or 50 to 60 grams if necessary to achieve and maintain a state of dietary ketosis. Keep in mind that physical activity plays a significant role. The more active you are, the more carbohydrates and fat you'll burn.

❏ Have at least six (6) protein servings a day (one each for breakfast, morning snack, lunch, afternoon snack, dinner, and evening snack). Choose foods from the Weight Loss Protein list and/or any of the

Lean for Life protein products. Each food choice or product selection equals one serving. *Depending on your current weight and level of activity, you may need more than six protein servings a day to control your hunger and maintain energy, up to a maximum of twelve (12) servings. Let your ketostick reading and how you're feeling be your guide. Never have fewer than six servings per day, however —you need the protein!*

❑ Use your Daily Action Plan to record each of your protein servings and how many carbohydrate grams they contain. Aim for a daily total of approximately 50 to 100 grams of carbohydrates, for ketosis.

❑ Take your Lean for Life vitamin/mineral supplements, or an equivalent, as directed on the label. Taking your vitamin supplement with a protein serving may help prevent the stomach upset some people experience when taking vitamins on an empty stomach. Storing your vitamins in the freezer may also help.

❑ Drink at least 80 ounces of water or other calorie-free beverages a day.

❑ Unless you have high blood pressure, you may add salt to your food during your Protein Days. If you tend to have lower blood pressure, the addition of salt may help alleviate the slight dizziness some dieters occasionally experience. (Please refer to page 25 for information about sodium and potassium.)

❑ Test for ketosis on the morning of your second Protein Day. When you first get out of bed, empty your bladder. Then, approximately 10 to 15 minutes later, before having a protein serving or drinking a large amount of fluid, test your urine with a ketostick, following the directions on the ketostick bottle label. If your ketostick shows a pink to purple color, you are in ketosis and can immediately begin the Weight Loss Menu Plan. Most people find it takes three full Protein Days to achieve "good color," so don't be discouraged. After a maximum of three Protein Days, move on to the Weight Loss Menu Plan regardless of the color on your ketostick (unless you are under medical supervision and directed to do otherwise). You will continue testing for ketosis every morning during Weight Loss.

❑ Beginning with your Protein Days and continuing throughout the Weight Loss module, we recommend taking a sugar-free daily fiber supplement. In addition to promoting bowel regularity, fiber has many other health benefits. A high fiber diet improves cholesterol, decreases the risk of developing colon cancer, and has been shown to play a role in the prevention of Type 2 diabetes. You may use an over-the-counter sugar-free fiber supplement of your choice, or one of the Lean for Life flavored fiber drinks.

"WHAT SHOULD I EAT ON MY PROTEIN DAYS?"

The choice is yours. With the variety of options available, you can enjoy a different menu on every one of your Protein Days. **During your Protein Days, choose only from the Protein list included in the "Food Choices, Servings, and Carbohydrate Counts" on page 37.** You may mix and match your choices for variety and convenience.

SAMPLE PROTEIN DAY MENU

You may use any of the Protein food selections or Lean for Life protein products, or "mix and match" them throughout the day for variety and convenience.

BREAKFAST
1 egg or 2 egg whites
     OR
1 Lean for Life Creamy Hot Cocoa

MORNING SNACK
2 ounces fat-free cheese
     OR
1 ounce Lean for Life Salted Soy Nuts

LUNCH
2 1/2 ounces water-packed tuna
     OR
1 Lean for Life Homestyle Chicken Soup with Noodles

AFTERNOON SNACK
4 ounces low-fat cottage cheese
     OR
1 Lean for Life Peanut Butter Bar

DINNER
3 1/2 ounces chicken or turkey breast
     OR
1 Lean for Life Savory Beef Soup with Vegetables

EVENING SNACK
2 1/2 ounces lean/fat-free cold cuts
     OR
1 Lean for Life Creamy Vanilla Shake

Note: You may need more than six protein servings to control hunger and maintain energy.

WHAT ARE LEAN FOR LIFE HIGH PROTEIN NUTRITIONAL PRODUCTS?

In addition to the many food choices included on the Protein food list on page 37, you may use any of the Lean for Life protein nutritional products during your program. These high protein, low carbohydrate, low calorie products have been specifically designed for use on all phases of the program and may be used as **the protein portion of meals, as a snack, and on Protein Days.**

While it's entirely realistic for you to succeed on the program without using any of the Lean for Life products mentioned in this book, they can enhance your experience by providing more of what this program is all about: choices. The Lean for Life product line offers dozens of options, ranging from only 1-16 grams of "usable" carbohydrate per serving. (See Counting Carbohydrates: "Usable" Carbs, on the following page, for more information.)

There's something for every appetite, including:

❏ **Protein Bars:** These delicious bars are available in a variety of flavors, including Chocolate Chip, Peanut Butter Crunch, Lemon Crisp, Double Chocolate, Chocolate Mint, Cinnamon Oatmeal Raisin, Creamy Coconut, and Apple Cobbler Crunch

❏ **Shakes and Puddings:** Choose from a selection of shakes in such flavors as Creamy Vanilla, Creamy Chocolate, and Pina Colada, and puddings such as Double Chocolate, Banana Cream, and Rice & Raisin

❏ **Fruit Flavored Cold Drinks:** Flavors like Peach-Mango, Wildberry Passion, and Orange are nutritious and delicious

❏ **Hot Drinks:** Creamy Hot Cocoa, Café Au Lait, Cappuccino, Irish Cream Hot Cocoa are among our bestselling hot drinks

❏ **Hot Soups:** Choose from such favorites as Homestyle Chicken with Noodles, Chicken Bouillon, Cream of Chicken with Vegetable, Beef with Vegetable, Cream of Tomato, Cream of Mushroom, and Asparagus

❏ **Hot Dishes:** Selection includes Old Time Chili, Spaghetti Bolegnese, Old Fashioned Oatmeal, and Scrambled Eggs

❏ **Soy Nuts:** A crunchy, salty snack treat

The Lean for Life product line is ever-changing. Updated product lists are available upon request by calling 1-800-LINDORA and by checking the "Products" page at www.leanforlife.com.

COUNTING CARBOHYDRATES: "USABLE" CARBS

Many of the Lean for Life products contain ingredients that are classified as carbohydrates but cannot be fully absorbed and "used" by the body. Even though these ingredients are not fully absorbed by the body, they must be included in the "total carbohydrate" number listed on the product's nutritional label. For example, the product label may show the "total carbohydrate" number as 21 grams while the number of carbohydrates your body actually "uses" may only be 16 grams.

We provide the "usable" carbohydrate number for every Lean for Life product. This is the number you'll write on your Daily Action Plan whenever you use a Lean for Life product. *The "usable" carb number applies to the Lean for Life products only – you will use the "total" carbohydrate number for all other products and foods.*

You'll find the usable carb count for all Lean for Life products listed on the Lean for Life Product Order sheet. The sheet is free and you can get a copy by calling 1-800-LINDORA. This information is also available at www.leanforlife.com. Simply click on "Products", then click on the name of the product for which you'd like more information.

WEIGHT LOSS MENU DAYS

After completing your Initial Protein Days, you'll move directly to the Weight Loss Menu Plan, with one Protein Day each week. During Weight Loss you'll be paying attention to the number of grams of carbohydrates in the food you choose, as well as how much and how often you're eating. You'll keep your daily carbohydrate intake somewhere within the range of 50 to 100 grams to maintain a fat-burning state of dietary ketosis.

On Weight Loss Menu Days, you'll be eating three meals and three protein snacks a day. The food selection on the Lean for Life Weight Loss menu is "limited" to provide the best weight loss and ketosis results. Foods that are not included among the menu choices may be too high in calories, carbohydrate and/or fat, and too low in protein. Foods that tend to "trigger" cravings and "binge" eating are also not included.

There is a strong cognitive (thinking process) restructuring component built into the program to provide long-term benefits as well as immediate results. In addition to helping you achieve your immediate weight loss goal, the Weight Loss menu is specifically designed to help you change the way you think about food and how you "use" it. The eating plan during this phase of the program builds a basis and beginning structure for the time when you achieve your weight goal and move on to the Lifetime Maintenance phase and add many more foods to your menu. It has been revised and refined over 30 years based on our clinical experience with many thousands of patients. For optimal results, we encourage you to resist the temptation to modify the food choices or meal and snack structure of the Menu Plan.

Your weekly Protein Day will follow the same guidelines you used during your three Initial Protein Days at the start of the program, except you'll do one day instead of three. Please read Your Weekly Protein Day on pages 40-41.

HOW TO DO YOUR MENU DAYS

❏ Eat three meals and three snacks a day. Follow the Weight Loss Menu Plan on page 36 and choose your foods from the lists on pages 37-39. Some people may need more than three snacks a day to control hunger and maintain energy, especially if active.

❏ Use your Daily Action Plan to write down *everything* you eat and drink, and how many carbohydrate grams each item contains.

❏ Drink at least 80 ounces of water or other calorie-free liquids a day.

❏ Take your Lean for Life vitamin/mineral supplement, or an equivalent, according to package directions, every day.

❏ Prepare foods without the use of oils or fats. Non-stick cooking sprays may be used lightly.

❏ Spices may be used, but avoid spice mixes that contain sugar.

❏ Do not combine meals or "save" foods to eat at another time. The meals are designed to provide an appropriate balance of protein, carbohydrates, and total calories to maintain ketosis, promote optimal weight loss, and reduce cravings. In addition, the Menu Plan is structured to help you develop intentional eating habits that will help you control your weight for life.

❏ Allow approximately 4 to 5 hours between meals, with protein snacks in-between. Active or larger individuals may need more than three snacks a day.

❏ Accurately weigh and measure all servings. Use the proper measuring tools such as a food scale, measuring cups and spoons. When using measuring cups and spoons, be sure to use "level" measurements for accuracy.

❏ If you would like to have more than one type of vegetable, fruit or protein at a meal, you may do so by combining partial portions to make a whole serving. For example, if you want bean sprouts and cabbage at the same meal, you will have a half-portion of each.

❏ Do not skip meals or eat less food; doing so may lower your metabolism, compromise your nutritional status, and trigger cravings.

❏ Unless you have high blood pressure, you may add table salt to your food. If you tend to have lower blood pressure, the addition of salt may help alleviate the slight dizziness some dieters occasionally experience.

Please review the information about sodium and potassium on pages 25-26 regarding symptoms of muscle weakness and/or cramps, fatigue or lack of energy, or dizziness.

❏ Check your ketostick every morning. Empty your bladder when you first get out of bed. Then, about 10 to 15 minutes later, before eating breakfast or drinking a large amount of fluid, test your urine with the ketostick, following the directions on the ketostick bottle.

If your ketostick shows a pink to purple color, you are in ketosis and will continue to follow the Menu Plan.

If your ketostick is negative for ketosis (a white or beige color), you have reverted back to using carbohydrates for energy instead of primarily burning your excess fat stores. Please read "If Your Ketostick Is Negative" on page 41 for information about what to do next.

❏ We recommend taking a daily sugar-free fiber supplement throughout the Weight Loss phase. In addition to promoting bowel regularity, fiber has many other health benefits. A high fiber diet improves cholesterol, decreases the risk of developing colon cancer, and has been shown to play a role in the prevention of Type 2 diabetes. You may use an over-the-counter sugar–free fiber supplement of your choice, or one of the Lean for Life flavored Fiber Drinks.

❏ Essential fatty acids serve important metabolic roles in providing the necessary building blocks for the body's normal growth, repair, and normal function. Because linoleic and alpha linoleic acids cannot be produced by the body, we recommend that you include a total of one ounce (two tablespoons) of safflower, flaxseed, soybean, or olive oil in your menu plan each week. Using one (1) *teaspoon* of oil a day when cooking, or as a salad dressing, six days a week, will provide the recommended one ounce per week. Do not exceed this amount or you may add too many calories and interfere with your weight loss results.

If you prefer not to use oil, you may take an essential fatty acid supplement in capsule form, as directed on the bottle. Do not use both the supplement and the oil in your food, as you may consume too many calories and interfere with your weight loss results.

YOUR WEIGHT LOSS MENU PLAN

Choose your foods from the Food Choices, Servings, and Carbohydrate Counts list on pages 37-39.

BREAKFAST
1 Protein
1 Fruit OR 1 Grain
Choice of any calorie-free beverage

MORNING SNACK
Choice of one serving from the Protein list.

LUNCH
1 Protein
1 Vegetable
1 Fruit
2 cups, torn lettuce**
Salad dressing: choice of any fat free product, up to 15 calories and 3 grams carbohydrate***
Choice of any calorie-free beverage

AFTERNOON SNACK
Choice of one serving from the Protein list.

DINNER
1 Protein
1 Vegetable
1 Fruit
2 cups, torn lettuce **
Salad dressing: choice of any fat free product, up to 15 calories and 3 grams carbohydrate***
Choice of any calorie-free beverage

EVENING SNACK
Choice of one serving from the Protein list.

MISCELLANEOUS
Your choice of one serving twice per day, with the meals of your choice:

Creamer (powdered)	1 tsp.
Gelatin (diet)	1/2 cup
Green onion (tops)	1 tsp.
Horseradish	1 tsp.
Jalapeno Pepper	2 small
Margarine (nonfat)	1 Tbsp. (5 cal. max)
Mustard	1 tsp.
Pimento	1 tsp.
Radishes	2 medium
Vinegar (unseasoned)	2 Tbsp.

BEVERAGES
Water
Coffee*
Decaffeinated coffee
Tea (hot or iced)*
Herbal tea
Diet soda*
Diet seltzer
Diet mineral water
Any other calorie-free drink

---

* This beverage may contain caffeine, which tends to stimulate appetite and may make you feel jumpy or "wired". If you choose drinks containing caffeine, you may want to limit them. If you reduce or eliminate caffeine, do it *gradually* to prevent withdrawal symptoms that often occur when stopping "cold turkey."

** Carbohydrate = 3 grams

*** Or you may use 1 tsp. olive, safflower, soybean, or flaxseed oil according to the guidelines on page 35.

FOOD CHOICES, SERVINGS, AND CARBOHYDRATE COUNTS

PROTEIN

Your choice of one serving each at *breakfast, morning snack, lunch, afternoon snack, dinner, and evening snack.* Be sure to weigh meat, seafood, and poultry (raw, skinned and boned), with all visible fat removed. Broil, boil, barbecue, microwave, roast, or "fry" in a nonstick pan using a nonfat, nonstick spray.

Food Choice	Serving Size	Carbohydrates Per Serving
Meat and Poultry Selections		
Beef heart (ground)	3½ oz.	3
Beef flank	"	0
Beef Sirloin (ground) 7% fat maximum	3 oz.	0
Beef round	3½ oz.	0
Chicken breast (fresh or frozen)	"	0
Chicken breast (canned white, water-packed)	2½ oz.	0
Cold cuts (97-98% lean/fat free)	2½ oz.	1
Pork Tenderloin (lean)	3 oz.	0
Turkey (white breast)	3½ oz.	0
Turkey breast (ground) 97% fat free	"	0
Veal	"	0
Dairy Selections		
Cheese (fat-free)	2 oz.	0
Cottage cheese (lowfat, plain)	4 oz.	4
Egg (limit if cholesterol is high or use EggBeaters)	1	1
Egg whites (no yolks)	2	1
Milk (nonfat)	1 cup	12
Yogurt (nonfat, plain)	½ cup	9

Lean for Life Protein Products

Lean for Life Protein products may be used as a protein serving. See page 32 for more information.

Food Choice	Serving Size	Carbohydrates Per Serving
Vegetarian Selections		
Tofu (fat-free)	6 oz	2
Veg-e-burger	⅓ cup	3
Veg-e-cutlet or meat substitute	No less than 15 grams of protein per serving	No more than 12 grams of carbohydrate per serving
Seafood Selections		
Catfish	3½ oz.	0
Cod	"	0
Crab	"	1
Haddock	3½ oz.	0
Halibut	"	0
Lobster	"	1
Orange roughy	"	0
Perch	"	0
Salmon	"	0
Scallops	"	2
Sea Bass	"	0
Shark	"	0
Shrimp	"	1
Snapper	"	0
Sole	"	0
Swordfish	"	0
Trout (Rainbow)	"	0
Tuna (white, fresh or frozen)	"	0
Tuna (canned white albacore, water-packed)	2½ oz.	0
Turbot	3½ oz.	0

GRAINS

Your *breakfast* menu includes your choice of either one serving of fruit *OR* one serving of grain from the following list:

Food Choice	Serving Size	Carbohydrates Per Serving	Food Choice	Serving Size	Carbohydrates Per Serving
Bread (whole grain, 80 calories or less)	1 slice	15	Nutri-Grain (Barley) (Corn)	³/₄ cup "	26 27
Cheerios	³/₄ cup	12	Nutri-Grain (Rye) (Wheat)	³/₄ cup "	25 28
Chex (Bran)	"	30	Oatmeal (cooked)	¹/₂ cup	12
(Corn)	"	19	Post Oat Flakes	³/₄ cup	21
(Rice)	"	19	Post Bran Flakes	³/₄ cup	23
(Wheat)	"	28	Product 19	"	21
Cream of Wheat (cooked)	¹/₂ cup	13	Rice Krispies	"	18
Cream of Rice	"	14	Shredded Wheat (or Wheat Bran)	"	23
Crispix	³/₄ cup	19			
Grapenut Flakes	"	17	Special K	³/₄ cup	16
Kashi (Puffed)	³/₄ cup	12	Team Flakes	"	27
Kellogg's 40+ (Bran Flakes)	"	23	Toasties	"	18
			Total (Wheat)	"	17
Life	"	24	(Corn)	"	18
Malt-O-Meal (cooked)	¹/₂ cup	13	Wheaties	"	18

VEGETABLES

Your choice of one serving each at *lunch* and *dinner*. Measure raw, frozen (thawed), water packed (drained), unless otherwise stated. No sugar added.

Food Choice	Serving Size	Carbohydrates Per Serving	Food Choice	Serving Size	Carbohydrates Per Serving
Asparagus	1 cup	8	Mushrooms, raw	2 cups	7
Bean sprouts	"	14	Okra	1 cup	8
Broccoli	"	5	Onion	¹/₂ cup	6
Cabbage	"	4	Pepper (red or green)	1 small	4
Carrots	¹/₂ cup	8			
Celery	1 cup	6	Spinach (raw)	2 cups	4
Chinese pea pods	"	11	(cooked)	1 cup	7
Cauliflower	"	5	String beans	"	8
Collard greens	1 cup	8	Sauerkraut	"	10
Cucumbers	"	3	Tomato	1 small	5
Jicama	¹/₂ cup	5	Zucchini	1 cup	4

FRUITS

Your choice of one serving each at *breakfast* (when not choosing a grain), *lunch* and *dinner*. Be sure your daily fruit choices include at least one citrus (indicated with a *). Choose fresh, frozen (thawed), or water packed (without sugar or fruit juice).

Food Choice	Serving Size	Carbohydrates Per Serving	Food Choice	Serving Size	Carbohydrates Per Serving
Apple	1, 2½" dia.	17	Kiwi	medium (3 oz.)	11
Applesauce (unsweetened)	½ cup	14	Mango	½ cup, sliced	14
			Nectarine	½ cup, sliced	8
Apricots (fresh)	2 medium	9	Orange*	1 small	14
(dried)	4 halves	9	Orange juice* (unsweetened)	4 oz.	12
Banana	½ small	13			
Blackberries	⅔ cup	12	Papaya	½ cup, cubed	7
Blueberries	"	14	Peach	1 small	10
Boysenberries	"	11	Pear (Bartlett)	½ small	13
Casaba melon	¼ (6½" dia.)	4	Persimmon	1	8
Cantaloupe	¼ (6" dia.)	11	Pineapple	½ cup, cubed	10
Cherries	10	11	Raisins	½ oz.	11
Dates	2	13	Raspberries	⅔ cup	10
Grapefruit*	½ small	10	Rhubarb	1 cup	7
Grapefruit juice*	4 oz.	11	Strawberries	1 cup	11
Honeydew melon	⅙ (6½" dia)	20	Tangerine*	1 (2½" dia.)	9
			Watermelon	½ cup, cubed	6

MISCELLANEOUS

Your choice of one serving, twice per day, with the meals of your choice.

Food Choice	Serving Size	Carbohydrates Per Serving	Food Choice	Serving Size	Carbohydrates Per Serving
Coffee creamer (non-dairy powdered, fat free)	1 tsp.	2	Margarine (nonfat, 5 cal max.)	1 Tbsp.	0
			Mustard	1 tsp.	0
Gelatin (diet)	½ cup	0	Peppers, jalapeño	2 small	2
Green onion (tops)	1 tsp.	0	Pimento	"	1
Horseradish	"	1	Radishes	2 medium	1
			Vinegar (unseasoned)	2 Tbsp.	2

YOUR WEEKLY PROTEIN DAY

Beginning with your second week of Weight Loss and continuing throughout your Lean for Life program, you'll choose one day each week as your Protein Day. Many people choose Monday, as it helps them get their week off to a great start and keeps them focused on their goal. With that in mind, the Lean for Life Program Overview on page 3 shows the first day of each week as a Protein Day. Choosing the same day each week makes it easy to remember so you can plan ahead and be prepared.

HOW TO DO YOUR WEEKLY PROTEIN DAYS

You will follow the same guidelines on your weekly Protein Day as you did for your three Initial Protein Days (pages 29-33) when you began Weight Loss, except you will do one day instead of three.

❏ You'll keep your carbohydrate intake somewhere in the range of 50-100 grams a day to maintain a state of ketosis. The exact number depends on the individual, so you'll need to experiment to determine the number that keeps you in ketosis. Keep in mind that physical activity plays a role. The more active you are, the more carbs and fat you'll burn. You'll know you're in ketosis if your ketostick shows a pink to purple color when you test your urine.

❏ Have at least six (6) protein servings a day (one each for breakfast, morning snack, lunch, afternoon snack, dinner and evening snack). Choose foods from the Weight Loss Protein list on page 37 and/or any of the Lean for Life protein products. Each selection equals one serving. Depending on your current weight and level of activity, you may need more than six protein servings a day to control hunger and maintain your energy, up to a maximum of twelve (12) servings. Let your ketostick reading, your weight loss, and how you're feeling be your guide. Never have fewer than six servings per day – you need the protein!

❏ Use your Daily Action Plan to record each protein serving and how many carbohydrate grams it contains. Aim for a daily total in the range of approximately 50 to 100 grams of carbohydrates, for ketosis.

❏ Take your Lean for Life vitamin/mineral supplement, or an equivalent, as directed on the label. Taking your vitamin supplement with a protein serving may help prevent the stomach upset some people experience when taking vitamins on an empty stomach. Storing your vitamins in the freezer may also help.

❏ Drink at least 80 ounces of water or other calorie-free beverages a day.

❏ Unless you have high blood pressure, you may add salt to your food during your Protein Days. If you tend to have lower blood pressure, the addition of salt may help alleviate the slight dizziness some dieters occasionally experience. Please read pages 25-26 for important information about sodium and potassium.

❏ On your Protein Days and throughout the entire Weight Loss module, we recommend taking a sugar-free daily fiber supplement. In addition to promoting bowel regularity, fiber has many other healthy benefits. A high fiber diet improves cholesterol, decreases the risk of developing colon cancer, and has been shown to play a role in the prevention of Type 2 diabetes. You may use an over-the-counter sugar-free fiber supplement of your choice, or one of the Lean for Life flavored fiber drinks.

WHAT TO DO IF YOU'RE NOT LOSING WEIGHT

In 1995, a six-month study of 6,032 Lindora clinic patients found that those who were in ketosis at least 90% of the time (during their Weight Loss weeks) and who recorded at least 25,000 pedometer steps per week, averaged a 3.2 pound weekly weight loss. Although weight loss results vary among individuals depending on factors such as age, gender, current weight, metabolism, activity level, and program compliance, you can probably expect to lose an average of two to three pounds a week. (You'll lose more during your first week on the program.)

Besides the scale, your ketostick is the most important tool you'll use to evaluate your Weight Loss program and determine your best course of action. If you encounter difficulty losing weight while on the program, check your ketostick result and carefully review the information on the following four pages.

IF YOUR KETOSTICK IS 'NEGATIVE'

If your ketostick reading is negative (white or beige) and you're not losing weight, or are losing very slowly, you'll know you've consumed too many carbohydrates and are primarily using carbohydrates for fuel instead of burning excess body fat.

Evaluate your carbohydrate intake from *everything* you're eating and drinking. The amount of carbohydrate intake that allows most people to achieve a state of ketosis is somewhere in the range of 50-100 grams a day. The exact number depends on the individual, so it is important to experiment and find the number that works for you.

Keep in mind that the more active you are, the more carbohydrates and fat you will burn. If you have a less active day you may find that you need to decrease your carbohydrate intake to stay in ketosis. You may go out of ketosis if you're less active but consume the same amount of carbs as you do on active days.

As you lose significant amounts of weight, you may find that you tolerate fewer carbohydrates to stay in ketosis. Decreasing your carbohydrate intake and/or increasing your activity level at this point can help.

Be sure to accurately measure *everything* you eat and drink; use measuring cups and spoons and 'level them off' across the top for accuracy. Keep an accurate record of *everything* you eat and drink on your Daily Action Plan. It all adds up – from "little nibbles" and "sips" to the "last bite" you ate from your child's plate while you were clearing the dinner table. Reading about Thelma's experience on page 101, and "Mr. Mito Says" on page 136 can help you become aware of how easy it is to misjudge what you consume.

You may be consuming more carbohydrates than you realize. You may have eaten a larger fruit portion, for example, and consumed more carbohydrates than you calculated. Or maybe you ate something that you thought was on the menu list — but wasn't.

You may be consuming more carbohydrates than you realize if you use sugarless items such as gum or breath mints. Products that contain less than one gram of carbohydrate per serving can legally declare "zero" carbohydrates on their label. Some of these items may contain 0.9 gram of carbohydrate, which can add up if you consume more than a couple of servings a day.

Recently, as this book is being written, there are a number of commercial protein products (such as protein bars) that have been found to contain more carbohydrates, less protein and more fat than their product label declares. While it's not mandatory that you use the Lean for Life protein products, we recommend that you use caution if using other protein product brands, and discontinue using them if your ketostick is negative or if you experience difficulty losing weight.

Since being in a state of dietary ketosis helps decrease hunger and cravings and helps you achieve optimal weight loss results, it's important get back into ketosis as quickly as possible. The best way to accomplish this is to immediately begin following the Protein Day guidelines until you're back in ketosis. This may take anywhere from several hours to a few days. Check your ketostick before each meal and return to the Menu Plan when you're back in ketosis. If you have completed three Protein Days and are still not in ketosis, return to the Weight Loss menu anyway and choose the lowest carbohydrate food choices until you are back in ketosis.

Increasing your activity level can help you get into ketosis. Take a longer walk or put extra energy into your exercise routine. And no matter what type of activity you participate in, the pedometer is a great tool to help you focus on and track fat-burning activity. If you regularly increase the number of steps you take each day—even throughout the normal course of your day—you'll increase fat burning. Focus on this *in addition to* any other type of exercise you do and you should notice a positive difference.

IF YOUR KETOSTICK IS 'POSITIVE' AND YOU ARE NOT LOSING WEIGHT

Your ketostick is 'positive' for ketosis if it shows a pink to purple color when you test your urine according to the package directions. There are several reasons why you may be consistently in ketosis and not losing weight, or losing weight slowly—or have even gained a pound or two. The following information will help you evaluate your program and take the appropriate action.

❏ Increasing your total caloric intake by adding items that are not included on the Menu Plan, or eating larger portions of the correct foods, may interfere with weight loss. Consuming too many calories, even if they are low in carbohydrates, can inhibit your weight loss even though you're in ketosis.

Keep in mind that "just a little" or "just a bite or sip" adds up faster than you may realize. Be sure to accurately weigh and measure *everything* you eat and drink and record it on your Daily Action Plan.

❏ Using items such as cooking oil, regular or low fat (instead of fat-free) butter or margarine, salad dressing, cheese, milk and other dairy foods that are not fat free will add calories that can interfere with weight loss. Be aware that oil and butter sprays are only "calorie-free" when used *very sparingly.*

When you limit your intake of carbohydrates, the body's next preference is to burn fat for energy. Adding extra dietary fat to your meals or snacks provides a source of fat for the body to burn instead of using your excess body fat for energy.

The body produces ketones from the dietary fat you eat as well as from stored body fat. That's why you can be in ketosis but not lose weight — because you're burning the fat you eat instead of your body fat! Following the low-fat Lean for Life Weight Loss Menu Plan ensures that your state of ketosis is from burning your excess body fat.

❑ If you've stopped losing weight even though you're in consistent ketosis and are following the Weight Loss Menu Plan correctly, please read Day 19 on pages 169-174 in the Lean for Life book about plateaus and how to work through them. Plateaus, which are a normal part of the weight loss process, usually occur sometime after your second week on the program.

To help "break" the plateau, you'll follow the Plateau Menu on page 172 for a maximum of three days. If you lose 1½ pounds or more before completing the three days, return to the regular Weight Loss menu.

Keep your weekly Protein Day as usual, even if it falls on what would have been a Plateau Menu day. Resume the Plateau Menu on the following day.

If your ketostick shows a white or beige color during this time, it means you've gone out of ketosis and should follow the guidelines on pages 41-42 for getting back into ketosis, instead of continuing the Plateau Menu.

❑ Fluid retention. There are many things that can cause temporary fluid retention such as hormonal changes; medication such as hormone replacement, birth control pills, steroids, and even some antibiotics; sunburn; sore muscles from over-exertion; lack of sleep; inadequate fluid intake (be sure to drink at least 80 oz. of water or other calorie-free liquids each day).

Some people believe that drinking water with lemon juice, or adding lemon juice to food, helps relieve fluid retention. Although there doesn't appear to be any scientific basis for this claim, many of our Lindora patients believe that it works for them. They cut a small fresh lemon and squeeze it into their water throughout the day. If you would like to try this, remember to write it on your Daily Action Plan and add six (6) grams of carbohydrate for the juice of a 2" lemon.

❑ Activity level. Attempting to lose weight without adequate physical activity can be very frustrating. Studies indicate that most dieters are not active enough to achieve effective weight loss. If you're having difficulty losing weight, we recommend that you "move more." Start slowly and increase your activity on a regular basis.

The body becomes accustomed to the amount and type of exercises you do, and after awhile you won't burn fat to the extent that you did when you first started exercising. At this point, you'll need to make your body work harder. Even if you consider yourself to be "active," it's necessary to modify your activity level as you become more fit and lose weight.

For example, if you walk for exercise you can increase your speed, distance, level of difficulty (include inclines, for example), and/or the frequency of your walks. Bend your arms at the elbow, swinging your arms as you walk. Try "interval training" — alternate periods of fast walking with short periods of slower walking during the same session. The closer you get to your lean weight, the harder you may have to work. Find activities that you enjoy so you'll want to participate in them frequently and with enthusiasm.

In addition, add short periods of exercise throughout the day whenever possible. Take the stairs instead of the elevator, "pace" while you talk on the phone instead of sitting, park farther from the door, get up to change the television channel instead of using the remote, and get out of your chair and move around during T.V. commercial breaks. Make a conscious effort to move quickly rather than at a slow or lethargic pace when engaging in normal activities throughout your day.

No matter what type of activity you engage in, the pedometer is a great tool to help you focus on increasing your fat-burning activity. If you regularly increase the number of steps you take every day (even throughout the normal course of your daily activity) you will increase fat burning. Focus on this in addition to any other type of exercise you do and you should notice a positive difference.

❏ Your mental attitude can affect how well you lose weight. Stress and depression tend to make it more difficult to lose weight. Make an effort to become involved in activities that are enjoyable and fulfilling. You'll find an excellent H.E.A.L.T.H. 'life model' on page 188 that can benefit you in many ways, in addition to helping you lose weight.

Medication is now available for the treatment of stress and depression. Consult your physician if you think you may benefit from using medication as you strive to integrate positive changes into your life.

PREP DAY 1

PREPARING FOR THE PROGRAM

*You'll learn how to effectively prepare
for the Weight Loss phase of the program.*

Before you begin the Weight Loss phase of the Lean for Life program, it's important that you prepare or "prep" for the next three days. The purpose of the Prep is to get your mind and body ready to accomplish your goal. Our clinic nurses tell us that patients who begin their program with a good Prep tend to feel better and achieve greater results during the Weight Loss phase of the program.

The Prep serves several purposes. It provides a comfortable transition into "dieting," especially for those whose eating habits have been undisciplined and unstructured. It also offers an opportunity for you to satisfy any lingering cravings before you begin the program.

If you've been dieting and restricting your calories for two weeks or more, the Prep can help replenish your body's reserves of essential fatty acids and amino acids. What's more, the Prep may be beneficial in helping to allow for gallbladder contraction. Research studies suggest there may be a small, temporary increased risk for the development of gallstones in overweight or obese individuals during weight loss. This appears to be related to the absence, over a period of time, of a small but necessary amount of fat in the diet that allows for gallbladder contraction. A good Prep helps provide that fat. Throughout the Weight Loss phase, you will also be eating foods that contain adequate but reduced amounts of fat, which help to reduce the risk of gallbladder disease.

If you have, or have had, any history that suggests gallbladder disease (attacks of sharp pain in your right upper abdomen, usually accompanied by nausea, gas and/or bloating after eating), be sure to discuss your symptoms with your doctor. It's important to be aware of the risks associated with weight loss and to carefully monitor any physical symptoms.

HOW TO PREP

1. During the three-day Prep, be sure to eat at least three complete meals a day. Your meals should include a protein food, a salad with dressing, a potato or other starch, vegetables, fresh fruit, and milk or the calorie-free beverage of your choice. Make sure your between-meal snacks are protein-based — foods such as cheese, nuts, seeds, celery with peanut butter, yogurt. Review the Sample "Prep Day" Menu on the following page for examples of food choices.

   If there are certain high fat foods you sometimes crave but try to avoid, such as pizza or cheeseburgers, for example, you may have them now. The Prep is not an excuse to "pig out," yet it is an opportunity to satisfy any nagging cravings before beginning the Weight Loss phase of the program. Do your best to avoid or limit candy, cakes, cookies, pies, and alcohol, as they can trigger cravings and stimulate your appetite. And use common sense. People who make the mistake of treating the three Prep Days as a "last hurrah" can end up unnecessarily gaining as much as 10 pounds. Why set the starting line back when you don't need to?

2. Begin taking your Lean for Life vitamin/mineral supplements (or an equivalent), every day as directed on the bottle.

3. Begin drinking 80 ounces of water or other calorie-free beverages a day. (Three 32-ounce squeezable sports bottles make it easy to remember how much water you're drinking.)

4. Continue with any exercise program you currently follow.

GETTING IT TOGETHER: YOUR RECIPE FOR SUCCESS

To prepare for the Weight Loss phase of the program, you'll need to gather these "ingredients" over the next few days. These items can be purchased at most drug or discount stores; many may be ordered through the Resources section of this book.

- ❏ Ketone strips (Fat Burning Indicators)
- ❏ Food scale
- ❏ Measuring cups and spoons
- ❏ Water bottle (30 oz. or larger)
- ❏ Weight scale
- ❏ Tape measure
- ❏ Pedometer (step counter)
- ❏ Cassette player
- ❏ Blank cassette tape
- ❏ Your food shopping list

SAMPLE "PREP DAY" DIET

BREAKFAST

2 eggs or omelette
Bacon, ham, or sausage (if desired)
1 slice whole wheat toast with butter
6-8 ounces unsweetened orange juice

LUNCH

Tuna salad sandwich, chicken salad sandwich,
    or pizza
Green salad with dressing
Fresh fruit
Coffee or any calorie-free beverage

DINNER

6 ounces steak or fish
Baked potato with butter and sour cream
Green salad with dressing
Fresh fruit or other dessert
Coffee or any calorie-free beverage

SNACKS

Cheese, nuts, seeds, celery with peanut butter,
    yogurt

Your Turn

You've made the decision. You're determined to make it happen—no matter what—and you're ready to create a Plan of Action. So now what? Take a few minutes to identify and prioritize your reasons for becoming Lean for Life.

The first challenge is to stay focused. This isn't always easy, because there may be a part of you that raises every possible excuse to keep you from facing the challenge of making changes.

It's important for you to identify your "urgency factor." What was the "final straw" that motivated you to lose weight this time? Often, it's a specific incident, comment, or personal observation that inspires us to make changes.

For Kathy, it was being asked when her baby was due—even though she wasn't pregnant. For Ben, it was having his daughter wonder why his face turned red and he breathed so hard every time he climbed the stairs. For Joan, it was the realization she had worn the same two outfits to work every day for nearly three weeks because all her other clothes no longer fit. What's *your* reason for choosing to make a change in your weight at this time?

Take a moment to complete the following statement:

I decided it was time to do something about my weight when

_____

_____

Now sit down with a stack of 3 x 5 note cards or small sheets of paper. On each card, jot down one benefit you'll enjoy after achieving your weight loss goal. How will losing weight enhance your self image? How will others see you? Will it benefit you at work? Make it less fatiguing to play with your kids? Here are a few ideas to help get you started:

> "I'll be proud of how I look."
> "I will feel more in control."
> "I could make love with the lights on."
> "I would be able to tuck my shirt in."
> "I'll be more active with my kids."
> "I can play tennis again."
> "I'll look terrific at the reunion."

After you've written down all the reasons you can think of, prioritize them. Move the cards around until you've clarified your top five reasons for losing weight, then list them on the following page.

MY PERSONAL MOTIVATORS: HOW I'LL BENEFIT BY BECOMING LEAN FOR LIFE

1. _____

   _____

2. _____

   _____

3. _____

   _____

4. _____

   _____

5. _____

   _____

   Copy the above list on three note cards or pieces of paper. Keep one copy in your purse or wallet. Put the second where you're sure to see it every morning—in your medicine chest, on your bathroom mirror, or in your underwear drawer. Keep the third in a desk drawer at the office, on your car dashboard, or in your gym bag. These reminders will help you stay focused on why you're investing the time and energy to lose weight.

   Review your Motivator cards daily. Before long, you'll memorize them and can use them to help yourself maneuver around the inevitable temptations that are sure to come up. When you feel like swinging by the bakery instead of the gym, for example, take a look at your card. Once you do, you'll be much more inclined to think twice and to say "Not so fast!" When you find yourself wondering, "What's wrong with a donut every now and then?" your card has the answer.

ANY QUESTIONS?

Q: *Tell me more about the three Prep Days. I always thought an ideal diet was low in fat.*

A: You're correct, and you'll return to low fat eating after the short Prep. These three days of relatively higher-fat intake help to ensure normal emptying of your gallbladder. This helps protect you from problems that can develop during periods of reduced calorie intake. IMPORTANT: Being overweight increases your risk of gallbladder disease. At the same time, dieting may exacerbate an existing gallbladder condition. If you experience abdominal pain, immediately contact your physician.

Q: *What effect will the three Prep Days have on my cholesterol?*

A: It will not have a permanent effect. If you normally avoid the kinds of higher-fat foods recommended for prepping, you may experience a minor, temporary increase in your blood cholesterol level. Over the course of the program, however, many people experience a healthy decrease of cholesterol as well as improved HDL (the "good cholesterol").

    Chronic high cholesterol can be a health risk. If you have a history of gallbladder or heart disease, consult your doctor before beginning the program to determine whether you're physically able to do the program and if the three Prep Days are necessary. It may be better for you to proceed directly to "Phase 1: Weight Loss."

Q: *I'm afraid I'll gain weight during the Prep. Will I?*

A: You may experience a slight weight gain during the Prep, but don't panic. If you follow the Prep guidelines correctly, the slight gain is most likely due to a temporary change in your blood volume and will immediately be lost during your three Initial Protein Days. You may not gain any weight if you avoid eating sugar, candy and pastries, and don't think of this as a "pig out" or "binge" time.

PREP DAY 2

MOTIVATING MEASUREMENTS

You'll discover the importance of setting goals and measuring your progress.

The first day of your Weight Loss phase of the program is just around the corner. But before you start, you need to ask yourself an important question: *"How much weight do I want to lose?"*

This question is one many overweight people would rather avoid. The more weight people need to lose, the more resistant they will generally be to declaring a specific long-term weight loss goal. Instead of saying, "I will become Lean for Life by losing X pounds," they often hedge their bets by saying they want to lose "some weight" or that they want to continue on the program until they "feel healthier" or "look better."

The problem with such vague goals is that it's virtually impossible to determine when you've succeeded. Is "some" weight 15 pounds or 50? Is "feeling healthier" being able to tie your shoes without being short of breath or is it taking a three-hour bike ride on a hot summer day and living to talk about it? Does "looking better" mean no longer feeling self-conscious in a pair of shorts or being able to wear your favorite jeans from college?

Be honest. How much would you like to weigh when you complete "Phase 1: Weight Loss"? If you could blink your eyes and magically transform yourself into a leaner, healthier you, how much would the "new you" weigh? The more clearly you state your goal, the more likely you'll be to achieve it. After all, if you don't know where you want to go, how will you know when you've arrived?

There are a number of ways to determine your "ideal" or "lean" weight. Hydrostatic (underwater) weighing is a highly accurate method for determining your body's composition of lean vs. fat, but it can be expensive and isn't widely available. In our clinics, we use an electrical impedance method that provides computerized calculations of lean weight, standard weight range measurements, and percentage of body fat. People who don't have access to these methods can go to a local gym to have a skinfold thickness test done with simple calipers.

Here are several common-sense measuring techniques you can use at home:

"Never let yesterday use up too much of today."

— Will Rogers

- ❏ **Weigh yourself.** Do you have any idea how much you weighed when you last felt good about your body? If so, a simple bathroom scale can help you estimate an appropriate body weight and monitor your progress.

- ❏ **The proverbial "Rule of Thumb."** Here's another way to establish an "ideal weight." Women: Start with 100 pounds and add five pounds for every inch above five feet. Men: Start at 106 pounds and add six pounds for every inch above five feet.

- ❏ **The pinch test. Stand up straight.** Using your right thumb and index finger, gently squeeze a fold of skin and underlying tissue four inches to the right of your navel. If you can pinch more than a one inch, guess what? You've got fat to spare.

- ❏ **Measure up.** Measure your chest, waist, lower abdomen, hips, and upper thigh. Jot down the numbers below. This is a useful way to monitor fat loss. You'll be doing it again later in the program.

Chest _____

Waist _____

Abdomen _____

Hips _____

Thigh _____

CHEST

WAIST

ABDOMEN

HIPS

THIGH

BODY MASS INDEX

Height	19	20	21	22	23	24	25	26	27	28	29	30	35	40
58"	91	96	100	105	110	115	119	124	129	134	138	143	167	191
59"	94	99	104	109	114	119	124	128	133	138	143	148	173	198
60"	97	102	107	112	118	123	128	133	138	143	148	153	179	204
61"	100	106	111	116	122	127	132	137	143	148	153	158	185	211
62"	104	109	115	120	126	131	136	142	147	153	158	164	191	218
63"	107	113	118	124	130	135	141	146	152	158	163	169	197	225
64"	110	116	122	128	134	140	145	151	157	163	169	174	204	232
65"	114	120	126	132	138	144	150	156	162	168	174	180	210	240
66"	118	124	130	136	142	148	155	161	167	173	179	186	216	247
67"	121	127	134	140	146	153	159	166	172	178	185	191	223	255
68"	125	131	138	144	151	158	164	171	177	184	190	197	230	262
69"	128	135	142	149	155	162	169	176	182	189	196	203	236	270
70"	132	139	146	153	160	167	174	181	188	195	202	207	243	278
71"	136	143	150	157	165	172	179	186	193	200	208	215	250	286
72"	140	147	154	162	169	177	184	191	199	206	213	221	258	294
73"	144	151	159	166	174	182	189	197	204	212	219	227	265	302
74"	148	155	163	171	179	186	194	202	210	218	225	233	272	311
75"	152	160	168	176	184	192	200	208	216	224	232	240	279	319
76"	156	164	172	180	189	197	205	213	221	230	238	246	287	328

Body Weight (In Pounds)

Find your height (in inches) in the left column. Read across to locate your current weight. Your BMI appears at the top of that column.

❑ ***Determine Your Body Mass Index.*** Your Body Mass Index (or BMI) is considered one of the best indicatiors of your risk for developing serious diseases such as stroke, heart disease, and diabetes. A BMI of about 22 is considered optimal for health. The National Institutes of Health considers a BMI of 25 or greater to be a risk. Individuals with a BMI of 25 to 29.9 are considered overweight, and individuals with a BMI of 30 or greater are considered obese.

❑ ***Consult your clothing.*** For some people, the snug fit of a favorite pair of pants or skirt is a sure sign it's time to drop a few pounds. If you have clothes that are a little tight around your chest, waist, hips, or thighs, pin a note with today's date on the garment and hang it back in your closet. Jot a reminder on your calendar to try it on again in two weeks and note your progress at that time.

❏ *Take a good look in the mirror.* You may find this one difficult, but it's important to do because it can be a real "reality check." Stand nude in front of a full-length mirror and study the image you see. Is this a body you would choose? Survey various areas. What improvements would you recognize as evidence of weight loss and improved fitness? This is a method you can repeat regularly, setting new goals as you progress.

Remember: Healthy improvement is what's important. It isn't necessary, and in fact may be psychologically unhealthy, to strive for physical "perfection."

❏ *Ask a trusted friend or loved one to help you with an assessment.* It's easy to see what we want to see and to avoid the truth. Ask a trusted friend or loved one to give you a candid assessment of your physical being. Do this only if you think the person can be objective and supportive while sharing these observations.

Be sure to try at least two of these measuring techniques. Then, it's "Your Turn."

DR. STAMPER

"It's entirely within your power to rethink, reprogram, and redefine the role food plays in your life. The Lean for Life program will show you how."

Your Turn

Establish your weight loss goal.

It's time! Based on what you've just read, take a few minutes to establish your long-term weight loss goal—not how much you want to weigh a week or a month from now, but what you'd ideally like to weigh. What would that number be if achieving it didn't require any effort, if you could simply wish it true? Your goal weight is probably right in that neighborhood. And on this program, you can achieve it—not by "wishing" it true, but by learning and applying the skills and strategies necessary for becoming and remaining Lean for Life.

My current BMI is _____.

My "Rule of Thumb" ideal weight is _____.

Today I weigh _____ pounds.

My goal weight is _____ pounds

To achieve this goal, I will lose _____ pounds.

YOUR PERSONAL SATISFACTION QUOTIENT

How you feel about your life—your work, your family, your relationships, your finances, your health, your body— impacts everything you think, say, and do. Are you physically energetic? Are you happy more often than sad? Do you get along with others? Do you like yourself? Circle the number that reflects how you feel about your life *at this moment:*

| 1 | 2 | 3 | 4 | 5 | 6 | 7 | 8 | 9 | 10 |

I've never been more unhappy.

I'm generally satisfied with my life.

My life is terrific!

We will revisit this question later in the program.

Another Lean for Life Success Story

THEN&NOW

"When I started the program, I said I wanted to lose 50 pounds. I was afraid to tell the truth—that I really wanted to lose 100—because it sounded overwhelming. Then I remembered one of my grandmother's favorite expressions. She used to say that the difference between involvement and commitment was never more obvious than with a bacon-and-egg breakfast. 'The chicken,' she would say, 'was involved, but the pig was committed!' It dawned on me that until I declared my true goal, I was merely involved. Once I did, I became committed, and it's made all the difference in the world. I've lost 87 pounds and I'm still going strong!"

— Rob

WHY WEIGH?

Does the idea of stepping on the scale send shivers down your spine? For some, weighing themselves ranks right up there with oral surgery, public speaking, and unexpected letters from the IRS.

But rather than thinking of the scale as judge and jury or some measure of your value as a person, remember what it really measures: how much your body weighs. It's a resource that provides valuable information you can't get any other way. It's a tool—nothing more, nothing less.

Just as an architect wouldn't think of designing a house before measuring the lot, why do a weight loss program without measuring your progress along the way?

PREP DAY 3

THE MIND–BODY CONNECTION

You'll discover how what happens in your mind affects what happens in your body—and vice versa.

Words can make you blush. Jokes can make you laugh. Movies can make you cry. Conversations can make you sweat. A card or call from that special someone can get your heart racing.

The connection between your mind and body is undeniable. The thoughts you think, the emotions you feel, the images you see, and the things you do all affect your behavior and your body chemistry. Likewise, your body chemistry and your behavior affect how you think, how you feel, your impressions of what you see, and what you do.

Only recently have scientists and researchers begun to understand how profound the mind-body connection is, and how you can intentionally use it to achieve specific goals such as weight loss.

Every page of this book reflects the power and potential of the mind-body connection. Our goal is to give you the tools that will make this connection work positively for you.

If you're feeling sorry for yourself, we'll encourage you to do things that will give you pleasure. If just thinking about exercise makes you tired, we'll help you learn to think about it differently. If you're feeling edgy, we'll offer ways to relax. If you're frustrated, we'll share success stories of others who've experienced the same feelings and have overcome them. If you're overwhelmed, we'll suggest ways to refocus your thoughts and energy.

Together we'll explore the importance of treating yourself well, clarifying goals, and cultivating an "achievement attitude." You'll become an effective problem solver, learn how to mentally rehearse being successful, and understand what you can do to change your body chemistry.

Our patients are often surprised to discover that many successful weight loss strategies can be learned. You can learn to control cravings, eat lean, and enjoy exercise. You can also learn to feel deserving of—and comfortable with—a more attractive, healthier body.

VISUALIZING YOUR SUCCESS

No matter how enthusiastic you are when you start the program, it's easy to lose momentum once the initial excitement fades. That's why it's vital to have a visual reminder of your goals.

Here are two ideas to help you succeed. Choose whichever appeals to you most or come up with your own motivational idea. Whatever you do, make sure it's a graphic reminder of why you're on the program.

1. *Find an "After" photograph of yourself.* You may have to dig through boxes or photo albums, but find a picture of yourself when you were leaner and healthier. Choose one that captures the physical image you want to project again.

   If you don't have photographs available, thumb through magazines and cut out images of people who look the way you would like to look. Be sure to focus on overall body image rather than the face or hairstyle. And whatever you do, be practical. Don't set yourself up with unrealistic expectations. Nothing can be more demoralizing than comparing yourself to an airbrushed, perfectly lighted image of an actor or model.

   Some people find it valuable to do this exercise with someone they trust to give them honest feedback as to what body type is realistic and appropriate.

2. *Create an "After" picture of yourself.* One woman who succeeded on the program came up with a clever way to visualize her leaner body. Alice asked her daughter to take several photographs of her wearing a one-piece swimsuit. She selected one of the pictures as her "Before" photo and used a second photo from the same session to create her "After" shot.

"What lies before you and what lies behind you are tiny matters compared to what lies within you."
— Ralph Waldo Emerson

Alice took a fine-line pen and outlined her leaner, healthier body shape on the photo. Using a pair of manicure scissors, she trimmed away the weight she was determined to lose. With a few snips, she had created an image that motivated her to pursue her goal.

It's your future. Picture it!

HOW STRONG IS THE MIND–BODY CONNECTION?

❑   Susan Everson, an epidemiologist at the Western Consortium for Public Health in Berkeley, California, and her colleagues have shown that men who are depressed die from heart disease, cancer, and other causes at higher than average rates.

❑   Neurologists at the National Institute of Mental Health have found that practicing a physical skill for just a few minutes a day alters the brain, dramatically increasing one's ability to perform the task. The more one practices a task, the more developed the relevant area of the brain becomes.

❑   Richard Restak, M.D., author of *Brainscapes*, reports numerous instances of behavior affecting brain structure. Blind people who study Braille, for example, develop a larger area of the brain assigned to the use of the left index finger, the finger that "reads" Braille text.

DAY 1

ACTION PLANNING

You will know, day by day, exactly what is working for you

Today's Eating Plan

Today is the first of your three Initial Protein Days. Follow the step-by-step guidelines on pages 29-33.

"**P**eople are always blaming their circumstances for what they are," observed Irish author and playwright George Bernard Shaw. "I don't believe in circumstances."

Shaw clearly had little patience for those who wallowed in inertia and indecision. He would have loved the Lean for Life program.

"The people who get on in this world," he observed, "are the people who get up and look for the circumstances they want, and if they can't find them, *make* them."

That's exactly what your Daily Action Plan supports you in doing: creating "circumstances" in which you can enhance your success by stacking the deck in your favor.

The Daily Action Plan is a simple, easy-to-keep record you'll complete every day while on the program. To make it convenient for you, a Daily Action Plan is included for each day of the program. As you get into the habit of maintaining your Daily Action Plan, you'll notice it provides insights and information that will help you stay focused and motivated.

Lean *for* Life®
DAILY ACTION PLAN

Week (A) 2   Day 11   Date 3/5

Time	Meal Plans	Serving Size	Carbs (grams)
7:00 AM	**Breakfast** (B)		(C)
	Protein EGG	1	1
	Fruit or Grain WHEAT BREAD	1 SLICE	13
	Beverage DECAF COFFEE	8 oz.	∅
	WATER	30 oz.	∅
10:30 AM	**Protein Snack**		
	FAT-FREE CHEESE	2 oz.	∅
12:30 pm	**Lunch**		
	Protein CANNED TUNA	2½ oz.	∅
	Vegetable TOMATO	1 SMALL	5
	Lettuce + 1 TBS DRESSING	2 C	3
	Fruit STRAWBERRIES	1 C	11
	Beverage WATER	8 oz.	∅
	Miscellaneous RADISHES	2	1
	WATER	30 oz.	∅
3:30 pm	**Protein Snack**		
	YOGURT PEANUT PROTEIN BAR	1	10
6:15 pm	**Dinner**		
	Protein CHICKEN BREAST	3½ oz.	∅
	Vegetable ASPARAGUS	1 C	8
	Lettuce + 1 TBS DRESSING	2 C	2
	Fruit UNSW. APPLESAUCE	½ C	14
	Beverage HERB TEA + WATER	10 oz.	∅
	Miscellaneous WATER	8 oz.	∅
	DIET GELATIN	½ C.	∅
8:45 pm	**Protein Snack**		
	NON-FAT MILK	1 C	12
		TOTAL	80 (D)

Keto Reading (E) MODERATE
Weight 167 (F)
Vitamins 2 AM (G) 2 Noon   2 PM
Fluids (H) 8, 30, 8, 30, 10, 8 = 94 oz.
Activities (I) 30 MINUTE WALK
20 LEG LIFTS
TAKE STAIRS AT WORK

Pedometer Steps (J) 7,554

WEEKLY BODY MEASUREMENTS (K)

Chest 38 ½   Hips 43
Waist 31 ¼   Thighs 25 ¼
Abdomen 38

SUCCESS LEARNING TOOLS (L)

Read pages # 108 ~ 114
Audio Tapes RELAXATION
Affirmation (M) I CREATE MY OWN JOY!
I LOVE EXERCISE!

Plan to Overcome Today's Obstacles:
(N)
TAKE PROTEIN BAR TO EAT DURING AFTERNOON
MEETING. AVOID THE SWEET ROLL TRAY.
DRINK 30 OZ. WATER MID-DAY.

Notes:
CALL DEBBIE TO ASK ABOUT
FRIDAY'S MENU. REQUEST
GRILLED CHICKEN, RAW VEGGIES,
FRUIT AND LETTUCE.
READ MOTIVATOR CARD BEFORE SLEEP!
STAY FOCUSED — IT'S WORKING!

CHOOSE ONE DAY EACH WEEK AS YOUR "PROTEIN DAY."

Let's take a line-by-line look at a sample Daily Action Plan sheet completed by Stephanie, who lost 62 pounds on the program.

A. Begin by filling out the date, week, and day of your program. Remember that the Weight Loss Module lasts up to 28 days, unless you are under medical supervision, in which case the length of your program will be determined by you and the medical staff.

B. Write down *everything* you eat and drink, *every time* you eat or drink. Many well-intentioned people are oblivious to what—and how much—they consume. Immediately after every meal and snack, jot down the time, what you ate, and how much. Don't wait. Studies show that the longer you wait, the more likely you'll be to make an error.

C. During the Weight Loss module, you will also keep track of how many grams of carbohydrates you're eating. *Before you eat anything during this phase, know how many carbohydrates it contains.*

D. At the end of the day, add up your total carbohydrate intake.

E. Check your ketone measuring strip or "ketostick" every morning. Record the result. If, on any morning during the Weight Loss phase, your ketostick doesn't show color, carefully review the previous day's Action Plan. Look for clues as to what bumped you out of ketosis. Check the number of carbohydrates you ate the previous day. If you take in too many carbs, you will go out of ketosis. Don't beat yourself up, but instead learn from your mistakes so you don't repeat them. Keeping an accurate written record allows you to monitor how many carbohydrates you consume throughout the day.

F. Weigh yourself every morning, ideally around the same time every day. Whenever possible, weigh the same way every day, nude and after emptying your bladder. Record your weight.

G. Be sure to take your Lean for Life vitamins and mineral supplements (or an equivalent) and check it off on your Daily Action Plan.

H. During the Weight Loss module, it's essential that you drink a minimum of 80 ounces of water or other calorie-free beverages every day. Water is preferable. Keep track of everything you drink and log it in.

I. Write down the exercise you do throughout the day.

J. When you start using a pedometer (step counter), which we'll discuss later, you'll be able to keep a record of the number of steps you've walked each day. Exercise and activity provide countless physical and psychological payoffs: they elevate your mood, boost your metabolism, improve your ability to burn fat for fuel, accelerate weight loss, tone and firm your body, and help you feel more relaxed and less hungry.

K. Refer to "Measure Up" on page 53.

L. You will be instructed on these aspects of the program throughout the book.

M. Every day, you'll want to write down one or two statements that you will repeat to yourself throughout the day. Begin these statements with the words "I am...", and fill in the blank by describing what you are ready to experience that day. For example, "I am enjoying my Lean for Life program," or "I am doing something that matters to me!" As you'll soon discover, these affirmations and the other mental training activities you'll be learning will become powerful tools to help you become lean and healthy. We'll be discussing affirmations in more detail on page 175.

N. Anticipate challenges. First thing every morning, review your schedule and consider any obstacles you expect to encounter during your day. What is your plan of action for overcoming that particular challenge? Write it down. Remember your plan and be ready to implement it.

As you begin using your Daily Action Plan, you'll notice certain patterns emerging. Many of these patterns will be positive, but others will not. The beauty of keeping a Daily Action Plan is that it provides you a wealth of information about what's working and what isn't.

There are 28 blank Daily Action Plans in the book (one for each day of Weight Loss) and 14 blank Daily Action Plans for the Metabolic Adjustment phase. If your health care professional has determined that it's appropriate to extend your weight loss beyond 28 days, you'll want to make copies of the Daily Action Plans for use later.

Knowledge is power. Your Daily Action Plan is a powerful resource that will help you stay aware and focused on achieving your goal.

Lean *for* Life®
DAILY ACTION PLAN

PROTEIN DAY

Week ___I___ Day ___I___ Date _____

Time	Meal Plans	Serving Size	(grams)
_____	**Breakfast**		
	Protein		
	Beverage		
	_____		
	_____		
	_____		
_____	**Protein Snack**		
	_____		
_____	**Lunch**		
	Protein		
	Beverage		
	_____		
	_____		
	_____		
	_____		
	_____		
_____	**Protein Snack**		
	_____		
_____	**Dinner**		
	Protein		
	Beverage		
	_____		
	_____		
	_____		
	_____		
	_____		
_____	**Protein Snack**		
		TOTAL	

Keto Reading _____
Weight _____
Vitamins   AM   Noon   PM
Fluids _____

Activities _____
_____
_____

Pedometer Steps _____

WEEKLY BODY MEASUREMENTS

Chest _____ Hips _____
Waist _____ Thighs _____
Abdomen _____

SUCCESS LEARNING TOOLS

Read pages # _____
Audio Tapes _____
Affirmation _____
_____

Plan to Overcome Today's Obstacles: _____
_____
_____
_____
_____
_____
_____

Notes: _____
_____
_____

TODAY IS YOUR FIRST PROTEIN DAY UNLESS OTHERWISE
DIRECTED BY YOUR HEALTH CARE PROFESSIONAL.

HAVE MORE THAN 6 PROTEIN SERVINGS AS NEEDED TO
CONTROL HUNGER AND MAINTAIN ENERGY.

DAY
2

Today's Eating Plan

Today is your second Protein Day. Follow the guidelines on pages 29-33.

THE SELF-SABOTAGE SHUFFLE

You will learn through awareness and action how to stop sabotaging yourself.

Congratulations. You're doing it! You're now beginning the second of your three Protein Days. Although it's unlikely you're already in ketosis, you may have started to notice that something different is happening to your body. You may have awakened this morning "feeling thinner," and there may be other ways in which you feel different physically. If you have any discomfort, know that it's only temporary. You may want to review the section titled "How Will I Feel While on the Program?" from page 22.

As you begin moving down this path you've chosen, now is the perfect time to take a look at some of the detours that might slow you down.

Most weight loss and self-improvement programs steer clear of addressing physical and psychological obstacles. At Lindora, however, we've learned from experience that the best way to turn obstacles into opportunities is to anticipate them and to develop strategies for overcoming them.

During the course of your program, any number of things could go wrong. You can't plan for the fender bender that could happen on your way home from work any more than you can control the random earthquake, flood, or hurricane that might temporarily disrupt your life. But since they're not under your control anyway, let's put these kinds of catastrophes into a box, label it "Uncontrollable Life Events," and store it out of sight and out of mind for now.

Let's focus instead on what you *can* control: what you put into your mouth every day. People often define this control too narrowly. They say things like: "Today's a lost cause—I've got a business meeting at an Italian restaurant," or "How am I supposed to eat on the program when I'm hosting a pizza party for my daughter's Girl Scout troop?"

There's no question that some challenges are tougher than others. Whenever possible, it's best to steer clear of potential problem situations during the Weight Loss phase of your program. If they're truly unavoidable, the task then becomes how to successfully navigate those choppy waters of temptation.

Each of us is ultimately responsible for our own actions. You have the ability to deal with the inevitable inconveniences and difficulties that are sure to occur while doing a program in which you're eating differently from the way you usually do.

The key word here is *differently*. Most of us find it tough to change our patterns and do things differently. Change isn't easy. Routines become a way of life. When we know what to expect, we don't have to think about it.

Attempts at change are most always met with some inner resistance. Sometimes, it's obvious when this is happening. Comments like "I'm tired of this—I want something else" or "I'm not walking in this weather. Those clouds are going to break loose any minute!" are sure signs you're struggling with the part of yourself that's determined to maintain the status quo.

Steve, a Lindora patient who lost 34 pounds in eight weeks, caught himself complaining one day that it just "wasn't fair" that he wouldn't be able to "pig out" at his softball league's year-end barbecue bash. Mid-sentence, Steve couldn't help but laugh. "Wow! I sound exactly like my 2-year-old when she throws a tantrum," he observed. "The only difference is that I don't hold my breath!"

Resistance isn't always verbalized. In fact, it often surfaces in more subtle ways. Here are just a few examples, shared by four Lindora patients:

"I went grocery shopping the other night without a list. I was also hungry, which only made matters worse. As I was unpacking the groceries, my husband came home and noticed a bag of chocolate cookies. If they weren't my favorite kind, I'd swear someone put them in my basket by mistake. I don't even remember taking them off the shelf."

— Judy

Lean *for* Life®
DAILY ACTION PLAN

PROTEIN DAY

Week ___1___   Day ___2___   Date _____

Time	Meal Plans	Serving Size	(grams)
_____	**Breakfast**		
	Protein		
	Beverage		
_____	**Protein Snack**		
_____	**Lunch**		
	Protein		
	Beverage		
_____	**Protein Snack**		
_____	**Dinner**		
	Protein		
	Beverage		
_____	**Protein Snack**		
		TOTAL	

Keto Reading _____
Weight _____
Vitamins   AM   Noon   PM
Fluids _____

Activities _____
_____
_____

Pedometer Steps _____

WEEKLY BODY MEASUREMENTS

Chest _____   Hips _____
Waist _____   Thighs _____
Abdomen _____

SUCCESS LEARNING TOOLS

Read pages # _____
Audio Tapes _____
Affirmation _____
_____

Plan to Overcome Today's Obstacles:
_____
_____
_____
_____
_____
_____

Notes:
_____
_____
_____
_____
_____

TODAY IS YOUR SECOND PROTEIN DAY UNLESS OTHERWISE
DIRECTED BY YOUR HEALTH CARE PROFESSIONAL.

HAVE MORE THAN 6 PROTEIN SERVINGS AS NEEDED TO
CONTROL HUNGER AND MAINTAIN ENERGY.

"I was making dinner for the kids last night, and before I knew it, I'd nibbled a whole hamburger bun. After I realized it, I just stood there thinking, 'How—and why—did *that* happen?'"

— John

"All day, I was looking forward to walking after work. It's been really chilly, just how I like it. But then my friends Viki and Patricia called. They were heading to the mall to check out a big sale on linens. I needed new bedding, so I met them there. I got a terrific deal on pillow cases, but I never did take my walk."

— Cassie

"I guess I should know better than to talk on the phone while I'm making dinner. Gary called to tell me about the committee meeting I missed last week. I was paying more attention to what he had to say than to my food. I didn't realize it until later when I was cleaning up, but I nearly doubled my serving sizes."

— Christopher

"Whether you think you can or think you can't, you're right."

—Henry Ford

Four different people facing four different challenges. Each had the opportunity to control the situation, yet sabotaged him- or herself by not thinking, not planning, and not being fully aware. Instead of evaluating the situation and making a choice that reflected their goal, each went temporarily blank. The result? In each case, the old habits re-emerged.

Whenever we ask people who are sabotaging themselves what they want to achieve, they inevitably insist that they want to lose weight. They want to become Lean for Life. So then why don't they "just do it"? If only it were that easy! No matter how committed a *part* of you is to losing weight, there's *another* part that is inevitably going to resist change. That's the voice that says, "C'mon, one little piece won't kill you" or "You deserve it—you've been good!"

On Day 12, you'll learn all about your personal "Inner Committee" and how you can decide which voice will wield the greatest influence. For now, it's important to understand that change requires a heightened

ANY QUESTIONS?

Q: *Will I be in ketosis today?*

A: Is your ketostick showing color yet? After just one full Protein Day, it's unlikely, but checking it is an important habit to develop. Continue following your Protein Day eating plan. And while you're at it, take a walk!

DO YOU HAVE "BODY IMAGE DEPRESSION?"

Do you think about the shape, strength, and/or size of your body on a daily basis? Do you wish you looked significantly different from the way you do today? Do you feel fat, no matter how much weight you lose or how much positive feedback you receive? Are you jealous of, or intimidated by, those you consider more attractive and fit? Do you often feel unattractive or self-conscious no matter what you wear? Do you ever attempt to hide your body from your intimate partner or avoid looking at yourself in the mirror?

These are just a few of the warning signs of "Body Image Depression," which clinical psychologist Ellen McGrath defines in her groundbreaking book, *When Feeling Bad Is Good* (Bantam Books, 1994), as "the negative feelings of shame, contempt, and disappointment in our bodies" that many of us—especially women—experience "as we attempt to live up to impossible cultural standards of physical perfection, beauty, sex appeal, youth, and fashion."

Women, McGrath suggests, are especially vulnerable to Body Image Depression. "We are conditioned from infancy to believe that the major source of our worth is how attractive we are to others, especially men," McGrath writes. "A disproportionate premium is placed on being beautiful, pretty, attractive, cute, and sexy... For a vast majority of women, beauty remains the primary currency of our value and worth."

The pressure to be physically perfect and remain forever young, McGrath believes, are two of the most consistent sources of depression among women.

"The depressing reality is that the cultural pressures for female perfection are so strong and pervasive that even if we resist or reject them, they still continue to haunt most of us."

In her book, McGrath offers a series of "Action Strategies" for overcoming Body Image Depression.

"It's important to see yourself as a problem solver rather than a victim," McGrath says. "Get active. Create your own definition of what's healthy and attractive. Talk with other women about how cultural standards have changed in recent years. Make a list of the women you most admire—it can be a liberating reminder that many of the world's most accomplished women are valued and respected more for their character, courage, and substance rather than for their degree of 'physical perfection'."

state of awareness of what you are doing. Pay close attention to your thoughts and actions by making a conscious effort to be aware.

By taking a close look at your self-sabotage strategies as they occur, you're bound to discover patterns. Do you slip more at the end of the day when you're tired? Are your defenses down when you're stressed, angry, or on deadline? Do you tend to lose your focus on weekends?

Recognizing these patterns will help you become more aware of your personal blind spots. Is there a way to pace yourself or build exercise into your day so that you don't feel so vulnerable at dinnertime? Can you come up with other ways of reacting to stress or anger? Can you structure your weekends so they're no longer a 48-hour excuse for "blowing it"?

This is a program that can do more than change your body. It can also change your life. In the process of changing your eating and exercise habits, you will discover things about yourself you never knew before. The self-awareness you'll gain during the coming weeks can serve you in every area of your life. By the time you've completed this program, you'll not only be leaner and healthier, you'll be better prepared than ever to turn obstacles into opportunities.

THE LANGUAGE OF SELF-SABOTAGE

Do you know who tells you the most important words you'll ever hear? You do. That little voice within your head, the one that talks to you hundreds of times every day, is an incredibly influential character.

What voice, you ask? You say you don't have one?

DR. STAMPER

"Motivation is a decision. Remind yourself several times every day why you've decided to become Lean for Life."

Another Lean for Life Success Story

"I've come to realize that the actions I take create the results I get. Someone once commented that the harder he worked, the luckier he got. It's true. If I really want something, I do everything within my power to make it happen. When I'm truly committed, no temptation is strong enough to get in my way. It's not always easy, but everything has a price. If this simple truth were as easy to swallow as pizza or pistachios, I wouldn't have spent the past 20 years wishing I weighed 20 pounds less."

THEN & NOW

—Rick

DR. STAMPER

"Losing weight—
and keeping it off—
has at least
as much to do
with what we put
in our minds as
what we put
in our mouths."

That's the voice I'm talking about! Your inner voice—the one that says, "Turn left at the next light" or "You forgot to give Mom a call"—has considerable impact on the way you live. While your inner voice generally does its best to help and protect you ("You'd better drive slower in this rain"), it's not a big fan of change. In fact, it can be downright stubborn.

Let's look at five of the most common self-sabotage patterns people fall into and the negative self-talk, or inner dialogue, that fuels them.

All or Nothing Thinkers tend to see the world in black and white. If their performance falls short of their expectations, they see themselves as failures. Kate, for example, lost 23 pounds on the program, but couldn't take pride in her accomplishment. Why? Because her goal was to lose 25 and she kept telling herself that she "would never make it."

Overgeneralizers zero in on a single negative event or experience as proof of failure. Three weeks into his program, when Adam hit a temporary plateau where he didn't lose any weight, his first inclination was to give up: "I *told* you it wouldn't work. I may as well quit right now!"

Labelers can be brutal, especially with themselves. When Heidi gained two pounds the week after being laid off from a job she loved, her assessment of the situation was especially harsh: "I'm a total loser. I'm unemployed and I'm fat!"

Doom-and-Gloomers discount their success by insisting that, for whatever reason, their achievements "don't count." They hold on to negative beliefs, even when they've been contradicted by positive experiences. When Rebecca achieved her goal of losing 45 pounds, she had trouble enjoying her achievement. Her first reaction: "I don't really see that much difference. And who knows if it'll stay off, anyway?"

Conclusion Jumpers make general statements that have no basis in fact. Gustavo was enthusiastic about beginning the program until he learned that activity was an essential part of the overall strategy. "I can't walk," he announced. "Walking cramps my legs up." When one of our clinic nurses asked when he last experienced leg cramps, Gustavo admitted he never had, but quickly added that he was "positive" he would. By jumping to this conclusion, he overlooked the obvious: that the 70 extra pounds he had been carrying for the past six years were much more punishing on his legs than a daily walk.

Later in the program, we'll discuss how you can change this kind of negative inner dialogue. But until you realize a problem exists, it's tough to overcome it. Over the next several days, make a point to listen to the messages you convey to yourself through words and thoughts. How often—and how easily—do you fall into these patterns? By recognizing these traps, you'll be less likely to fall victim to them in the future.

MODERATE EXERCISE AND THE MAGICAL MITOCHONDRIA

Today's Eating Plan

Are you in ketosis? If not, plan to make this your third Protein Day. If you are in ketosis, you may begin the Weight Loss Menu Plan according to the guidelines on pages 33-39.

You can exercise more moderately than you thought and still lose fat.

D id you know you can burn fat by exercising *moderately?* Many people still believe that for exercise to make a difference, it has to be exhausting. For years, "No Pain, No Gain" was the anthem of the active. We were led to believe that unless our hearts were racing, our breath was short, and we ended our workout drenched, we had somehow shortchanged ourselves.

WHEN LESS IS MORE

In fact, the opposite is true. Doctors, health researchers, and fitness experts now know that a consistent program of moderate exercise is ultimately the safest, most effective approach for achieving and maintaining good health.

In March 1993, an expert panel was assembled by the American College of Sports Medicine and the U.S. Centers for Disease Control and Prevention, in conjunction with the President's Council on Physical Fitness and Sports. Concluding that only 22% of American adults are getting enough exercise, the panel speculated that "previous public

"The body you have at 20 depends on your genes, but the body you have at 40, 60, or 80 is the body you deserve, the body that reflects your behavior."

—Harvey Simon, M.D.

health efforts to promote physical activity have overemphasized the importance of high-intensity exercise."

Moderate exercise, such as walking, is now the accepted approach in exercise and fitness training. What qualifies as "moderate"? Any continuous movement of your hips and knees that causes you to exert yourself without becoming breathless. If, while exercising, you can't talk without feeling short of breath, slow down: it's not moderate enough.

In addition to being easier to do and less likely to cause injury than more vigorous exercise, moderate exercise has been proven to be the most effective way to increase the amount of mitochondria in your body.

MITO-WHAT?

Mitochondria. They're the tiny, egg-shaped structures in your cells that serve as fat-burning furnaces. Too small to be seen with an ordinary microscope, there are trillions in every human body. The more mitochondrial surface you have in your cells, the easier it is for your body to burn stored fat for fuel. If you want to burn more body fat, you need to increase the mitochondrial surface in your cells.

How can you do this? By increasing the amount of moderate exercise you do every day, you will increase the mitochondria in your muscle cells. The result? It'll be easier for your body to burn stored fat for fuel.

Increased amount of moderate exercise ➡ Increased amount of mitochondrial surface ➡ Increased ability to use stored fat for fuel

MEET MR. MITO

At Lindora, we encourage our patients to become "Mitochondriacs." We even developed a mascot to help remind them that movement matters. We call him "Mr. Mito." You've already seen his picture on your Daily Action Plan, and you'll be seeing more of him in the coming weeks. Think of him as your personal exercise and activity coach. He'll help you increase your daily activity level by reminding you to "Step It Up!" and showing you how to "exercise" without having to find an extra hour in your busy day. He'll have plenty of tips to share with you throughout the book.

Another Lean for Life Success Story

"I remember when I first received my pedometer and was encouraged to walk at least 10,000 steps a day. I thought to myself, 'Yeah, right!' I could barely walk to the bathroom. For the first few months, I only logged about 2,000 steps a day. But as my weight dropped, I've been able to walk more. I'm down 120 pounds and I often do 10,000 steps in a day."

— *Marsha*

HOW MUCH MODERATE EXERCISE DOES IT TAKE?

You don't have to devote a big block of time to exercise. Four 15-minute walks distributed throughout your day can be just as productive as a continuous hour of exercise. For most people, adding 30 to 45 minutes of moderate activity every day will do the job. Remember: *The more mitochondria you have, the more easily your body can burn body fat for fuel.* As it becomes easier to use up excess body fat, you'll lose weight more rapidly, move more easily, feel healthier, and become leaner.

Researchers at the University of Pittsburgh recently completed a study of 56 sedentary, overweight women. Each began walking and/or cycling five times a week for 40 minutes. Half of the women worked out continuously for 40 minutes; the other half divided their daily exercise into four 10-minute sessions.

After 20 weeks, both groups had boosted their aerobic capacity. But there was a significant difference. Not only did the women who exercised more often but for shorter periods adhere better to their exercise schedules, they also lost more weight.

It's important to create a schedule that works for you—one that allows time to do whatever exercise you plan for the day, whether in long or short sessions.

Why not take a 15-minute walk right now? Let yourself be pleased. Let yourself get moving. Feel the difference!

Lean *for* Life®
DAILY ACTION PLAN

PROTEIN DAY

Week ___**1**___   Day ___**3**___   Date _____

Time	Meal Plans	Serving Size	(grams)
_____	**Breakfast**		
	Protein		
	Beverage		
	_____		
	_____		
	_____		
_____	**Protein Snack**		
	_____		
_____	**Lunch**		
	Protein		
	Beverage		
	_____		
	_____		
	_____		
	_____		
_____	**Protein Snack**		
	_____		
_____	**Dinner**		
	Protein		
	Beverage		
	_____		
	_____		
	_____		
	_____		
_____	**Protein Snack**		
	_____		
		TOTAL	

Keto Reading _____
Weight _____
Vitamins   AM   Noon   PM
Fluids _____

Activities _____
_____
_____

\# Pedometer Steps _____

WEEKLY BODY MEASUREMENTS

Chest _____   Hips _____
Waist _____   Thighs _____
Abdomen _____

SUCCESS LEARNING TOOLS

Read pages # _____
Audio Tapes _____
Affirmation _____
_____
_____

Plan to Overcome Today's Obstacles:
_____
_____
_____
_____
_____
_____

Notes:
_____
_____
_____
_____

TODAY IS YOUR THIRD PROTEIN DAY UNLESS OTHERWISE
DIRECTED BY YOUR HEALTH CARE PROFESSIONAL.

HAVE MORE THAN 6 PROTEIN SERVINGS AS NEEDED TO
CONTROL HUNGER AND MAINTAIN ENERGY.

STEP IT UP!

How much exercise did you do yesterday? What did you eat?

You can answer these questions because you're maintaining a Daily Action Plan. But most people have no clue as to how many calories they consume, how many steps they've taken, or how many additional calories they've burned through exercise and activity on a given day.

As reported in the *New England Journal of Medicine*, people consistently *underestimate* the number of calories they consume and *overestimate* the number of minutes they exercise. That's why it's important to have objective measurements of food intake and exercise.

Your Daily Action Plan is your tool for monitoring your food intake. A pedometer or step counter is an easy way to monitor your physical activity and daily exercise. You can purchase pedometers at most sporting goods or discount stores. Information on the Lean for Life pedometer/step counter may be found in the Resources Section.

Once you have your pedometer, you'll clip it on your belt, waistband, or shoe every morning and record the number of steps you take on your Daily Action Plan before you go to bed.

Most Lindora patients aim for achieving 10,000 steps a day. If you haven't been very active, it may take time to work up to that many steps. I've been wearing a pedometer nearly every day for three years. When I first started wearing it, I considered myself to be a fairly active person. I've always tried to take the stairs instead of elevators and I often walk around my office while I'm talking on the phone. My daughter, who was just one year old at the time, had just started walking, and keeping up with her seemed like a nonstop workout.

I was shocked to discover that I was only logging about 3,500 steps a day on my pedometer! I thought of myself as active, but I was almost a couch potato. That's when I made a conscious decision to become more active. I now check my pedometer several times a day. If the number is low and it looks like I won't make my goal of 8,000 to 10,000 steps for the day, I either take a 10-minute walk or stand at my desk and shift my weight from foot to foot for five or 10 minutes while I continue to work.

A pedometer not only measures steps, but it also reminds you to take those steps. After you wear a pedometer for a while, you, too, will come up with different ways to make sure you get the activity you need to become leaner and healthier.

Aim for success, not perfection. Make it your goal to gradually increase your number of steps—then see, feel, and record your progress.

"The future belongs to those who believe in the beauty of their dreams."

— Eleanor Roosevelt

THE BENEFITS OF MODERATE EXERCISE

People who engage in moderate exercise on a regular basis enjoy such benefits as:

- ❏ Increased ease and maintenance of weight loss
- ❏ Increased metabolic rate
- ❏ Increased ability to burn body fat for fuel
- ❏ Increased responsiveness to insulin
- ❏ Increased strength, flexibility, suppleness, and stability
- ❏ Increased balance, agility, and coordination
- ❏ Increased enjoyment of physical activity
- ❏ Relief from anxiety
- ❏ Control over depression
- ❏ Improved sleep
- ❏ Stimulation of circulation
- ❏ Normalization of appetite
- ❏ Lower blood pressure
- ❏ Improved lipid and carbohydrate metabolism
- ❏ Improved appearance

ANY QUESTIONS?

Q: *Eighty ounces of water a day? I'll float away! Why is drinking so much water important?*

A: Water cleanses your system, curbs appetite, reduces fluid retention, keeps the urinary tract healthy, and helps prevent constipation. It flushes out the toxic chemicals used in agriculture, such as organophosphates, that have been stored in the body fat and are released into the bloodstream as the fat is being burned.

Drinking water can also increase your energy level. The slight dehydration that occurs when you don't consume enough fluid throughout the day can cause you to feel less energetic and become more easily fatigued.

Adequate fluid intake is necessary for the body to function properly, and the body fluid that's released throughout the day must be relaced in sufficient amounts. Your need for fluid replacement is increased during times of greater fluid loss as when you're in ketosis and during exercise.

WALKING OFF CALORIES

Find your current weight in the left column. The columns to the right itemize the number of calories burned based on the number of minutes walked.

Current Weight	Minutes Walked							Current Weight	Minutes Walked						
	5	10	15	20	30	45	60		5	10	15	20	30	45	60
110	20	39	61	79	114	166	225	215	36	72	108	144	216	324	432
115	20	40	63	82	118	169	234	220	37	74	111	148	222	333	444
120	20	42	65	85	123	176	245	225	38	75	113	150	225	338	450
125	21	43	66	87	127	185	254	230	39	77	116	154	231	347	462
130	22	44	68	89	132	191	264	235	40	79	119	158	237	356	474
135	23	45	69	92	136	201	274	240	40	80	120	160	240	360	480
140	24	47	71	94	141	212	282	245	41	82	123	164	246	369	492
145	24	49	74	98	147	221	294	250	42	84	126	168	252	378	504
150	25	50	75	100	150	225	300	255	43	85	128	170	255	383	510
155	26	52	78	104	156	234	312	260	44	87	131	174	261	392	522
160	27	54	81	108	162	243	324	265	45	89	134	178	267	401	532
165	28	55	83	110	165	248	330	270	45	90	135	180	270	405	540
170	29	57	86	114	171	257	342	275	46	92	138	184	276	414	552
175	30	59	89	118	177	266	354	280	47	94	141	188	282	423	564
180	30	60	90	120	180	270	360	285	48	95	143	190	285	428	571
185	31	62	93	124	186	279	372	290	49	97	146	194	291	437	582
190	32	64	96	128	192	288	384	295	50	99	149	198	297	446	594
195	33	65	98	130	195	293	390	300	50	100	150	200	300	450	600
200	34	67	101	134	201	302	402	305	51	101	155	205	305	460	612
205	35	69	104	138	207	311	414	310	52	103	157	207	310	467	623
210	35	70	105	140	210	315	420	315	53	105	158	210	315	475	631

Calculations based on walking three miles per hour and are rounded to the nearest whole number.

DAY 4

Today's Eating Plan

Today through Day 28, you'll follow the Weight Loss Menu Plan guidelines on pages 33-39, and do a Weekly Protein Day according to the guidelines on pages 40-41. If you go out of ketosis or experience difficulty losing, you'll follow the guidelines on pages 41-45.

THOSE @#%&*! CRAVINGS

You can learn to deal effectively with the physical causes of cravings.

You're having a terrific day. You feel focused, positive, and in control. You've exercised and you're eating well. Then suddenly, without warning, it happens. A nagging temptation for one of your favorite foods grabs hold and refuses to let go. The more you try to ignore it, the more tormenting it becomes. You feel lightheaded, irritable, edgy. Your mouth waters. Minute by minute, your willpower erodes like a sandcastle at high tide.

Welcome to the world of cravings, where powerful forces stronger than mere willpower rule. Cravings can be your worst nightmare, undermining your self-esteem, shaking your self-confidence, and derailing your weight loss program.

Cravings don't just happen. They're the result of various physical, psychological, and environmental factors that affect the way your body and brain function. Once you understand what causes them and how you can neutralize their impact, you'll have jumped a major hurdle on your journey to becoming Lean for Life.

One of the most common physical causes of cravings is an elevated "setpoint." If you just felt your eyes glazing over at the thought of reading "scientific stuff," stay with me. Cravings can be deadly to your weight loss efforts, so anything you can learn—and do—to counter them will stack the deck in your favor.

YOUR SETPOINT AND HOW IT WORKS

The human body was designed to store fat and then burn it as fuel. Your body is an exquisitely designed machine, in which millions of cells function in perfect synchronicity. Your brain, digestive tract, muscles and fat all work together through a highly complex system of biochemical feedback loops to maintain a stable weight. In other words, these different parts of the body "talk" to each other, coordinating their efforts to maintain a stable weight. That particular weight, which your body strives to maintain, is commonly known as the "setpoint."

Think of your setpoint as a thermostat. Just as a thermostat works to maintain a constant temperature by regulating the heating or cooling system in response to outside conditions, the setpoint raises or lowers your appetite and metabolism—the rate at which your body burns calories—in response to how much you're eating.

This raises an obvious question. "If my body's designed to maintain a stable weight," you may be wondering, "why did I gain weight in the first place and why is it so #*@&%! hard to lose it?" Here's the deal. If you live in the desert and the temperature outside is 85 degrees, your home's cooling system will have no problem maintaining an indoor temperature of 72 degrees. But if it's a sweltering 120 degrees outside, the cooling system will eventually become overtaxed. It won't be able to function adequately, so it will start maintaining the indoor temperature at higher than 72 degrees.

In essence, the same is true with your body. If you eat more calories and/or get too little exercise over a long enough period of time, your body's weight regulation system won't be able to cope adequately. It will adjust upward and your body's systems will "settle in" to support a higher weight.

So what happens when you start to lose weight? Because your body strives for equilibrium, its metabolic alarm system goes off as soon as you stop eating as much as you normally do. Your body demands food. Like the ravenous, man-eating plant in *Little Shop of Horrors*, it has one thing on its mind: "Feed me! Feed me!" You begin feeling uncomfortable, anxious, perhaps even edgy. The quickest form of relief? That's right—food! And thus, the cycle of losing and regaining continues.

DR. STAMPER

"There are many benefits to remaining in ketosis. One of the greatest is a dramatic reduction in hunger. You'll eat less because you'll want less."

Dr. Stamper has told patients for years that dieters don't fail because of a lack of willpower—they fail because of cravings. As long as your setpoint remains elevated, you will crave food whenever your body senses you're not eating enough to maintain your present weight.

As you can imagine, these mental "hunger alarms" make it especially difficult for overweight people to lose weight—and even tougher for them to keep it off. Your body will fight to hold on to whatever excess fat it has become accustomed to. It will also do its best to replace any weight you happen to lose. That's why it's essential to understand the nature of your food cravings and how to control them.

SO WHAT'S THE SOLUTION?

Here are three powerful short-term tools for immediate relief from the physical causes of cravings, as well as a fourth that yields both short-term and long-term benefits:

1. Since you'll be limiting your carbohydrates during the Weight Loss module of the program, your body will be using your stored fat as its primary fuel source. Throughout the program we'll refer to the physiological state of burning fat as "ketosis." Two of the benefits of being in ketosis are a dramatic reduction in hunger and fewer cravings.

2. Serotonin is a powerful neurotransmitter that regulates mood, hunger, and eating behavior. Low or fluctuating serotonin levels contribute to the urge to overeat—especially carbohydrates. Medications that elevate serotonin levels can help control the food cravings that result when serotonin is low. Consult your physician to determine whether such medication may help you.

3. When stressed, many people use food as a "tranquilizer." Although you may temporarily feel better when you do, the long-term results of using food as a coping mechanism can be disasterous. Stress management tools, such as mental training exercises, a 15-minute walk and the neck massage technique you'll learn later next week all help provide immediate relief from cravings by naturally modifying your biochemistry.

4. The moderate exercise strategies we discussed yesterday help decrease food cravings and benefit your muscle cells in two important ways. First, you develop more mitochrondria in your muscles through moderate exercise, which increases your ability to burn fat. You also develop more insulin receptors on the surface of the cells, which improves your body's ability to move sugar from the bloodstream into your muscle cells. This helps to stabilize blood sugar levels, which in turn lessens cravings.

Tomorrow, we'll explore another cause of cravings to see how people, places, and events can stimulate your food cravings—and what you can do to stay focused and in control.

Another Lean for Life Success Story

"My food cravings used to be relentless. I've made more midnight runs to the market than I care to admit. One night I was in line at a convenience store behind a guy who was buying a pint of vodka. His hands were trembling, and I remember feeling pity for him. Then it dawned on me that we really weren't that different. After all, I had gotten out of bed in the middle of the night to buy a pint of my own— double fudge brownie ice cream. Now that I've done the Lean for Life program, I experience cravings a lot less often. And when I do, I know what to do about it."

—Jody

PRODUCT LABELING: DO THE MATH

It was recently reported that some protein nutrition products contained far more carbohydrate than their labels declared. How can you avoid the consequences of inaccurate product labeling? Do the math—it's easy!

First, you need to know that there are 4 calories in one gram of protein, 4 calories in one gram of carbohydrate, and 9 calories in one gram of fat. Now, look at the product label and multiply the number of fat grams by 9, and the number of protein grams by 4. Add the numbers together and then subtract that figure from the total calories listed for the product. This will give you the number of calories that come from carbohydrates. Now divide that number by 4 (the number of calories in one gram of carbohydrate) and compare this figure to the carbohydrate grams on the product label. It should be equal to, or less than, the number of grams listed on the label. A higher number indicates there may be more carbohydrate in the product than the label declares.

KETOSIS + EXERCISE = INCREASED WEIGHT LOSS

The more you're in ketosis and the more steps you take, the more weight you can expect to lose.

That's the finding of a 1995 research project conducted by Jan Hunter, R.N., Lindora's former Director of Nursing Services and Clinic Operations; Jayme Davidson, R.N.; Deena Eshom, L.V.N.; Vickie Flatt, L.V.N.; and Carolyn Lehm, R.N.

The six-month study of 6,032 Lindora patients found that:

...those who were in ketosis more than 90% of the time—and recorded more than 25,000 steps per week—averaged a 3.2 pound weekly weight loss, while participants who were in ketosis less than 60% of the time—and logged less than 25,000 steps per week— averaged a 1.9 pound weekly weight loss.

The bottom line? Participants who were in ketosis more than 90% of the time— and averaged 25,000 or more steps per week—*lost 60% more weight* than those who logged fewer than 25,000 and were in ketosis less than 60% of the time. To maximize your weight loss results, stay in ketosis and keep moving!

WHY WALK?

When you walk, you:

- ❏ Improve your fat-burning capacity

- ❏ Improve your carbohydrate metabolism (increased insulin receptors)

- ❏ Improve your cardiovascular fitness (enhance circulation, heart and lung function, delivery of blood and oxygen to cells)

- ❏ Improve your mood (endorphins, your body's "feel-good" chemical, are released)

- ❏ Improve stress resilience (your ability to offset effects of stress hormones)

- ❏ Improve your ability to enjoy solitude

- ❏ Provide time for yourself to reflect, ponder and think

Lean *for* Life®
DAILY ACTION PLAN

Week _____ Day _____ Date _____

Time	Meal Plans	Serving Size	(grams)
_____	**Breakfast**		
	Protein		
	Fruit or Grain		
	Beverage		
	_____		
	_____		
_____	**Protein Snack**		
	_____		
_____	**Lunch**		
	Protein		
	Vegetable		
	Lettuce		
	Fruit		
	Beverage		
	Miscellaneous		
_____	**Protein Snack**		
	_____		
_____	**Dinner**		
	Protein		
	Vegetable		
	Lettuce		
	Fruit		
	Beverage		
	Miscellaneous		
	_____		
	_____		
_____	**Protein Snack**		
	_____		
		TOTAL	

Keto Reading _____
Weight _____
Vitamins   AM   Noon   PM
Fluids _____

Activities _____
_____
_____

Pedometer Steps _____

WEEKLY BODY MEASUREMENTS

Chest _____ Hips _____
Waist _____ Thighs _____
Abdomen _____

SUCCESS LEARNING TOOLS

Read pages # _____
Audio Tapes _____
Affirmation _____
_____

Plan to Overcome Today's Obstacles:
_____
_____
_____
_____
_____
_____
_____

Notes:
_____
_____
_____
_____
_____

CHOOSE ONE DAY EACH WEEK AS YOUR "PROTEIN DAY."

STOP!

Whenever you're tempted to do anything that might interfere with your program, **STOP**:

Stop! Visualize a stop sign and hear the word "stop." Immediately stop what you're doing!

Take a deep, cleansing breath. This creates a "window of opportunity" during which you can become aware of the temptation you're facing and can start over.

Observe your situation, yourself, and your options. What's going on? How are you feeling? Are you hungry, angry, lonely, tired? What are you wanting? What are you needing? What really matters to you? What choices do you have? What actions will help you move toward what's really important to you?

Plan of Action. Choose a Plan of Action based on one or more of the options available to you and put that plan into operation. Shift the focus away from food by doing something: taking a walk, calling a friend, sitting quietly for five minutes and letting your attention rest on your breathing, going window shopping, listening to music, working on a project, or reviewing your Motivator cards to remind yourself why becoming Lean for Life is important to you.

If you find yourself thinking "I'm tired of not eating what I want—I'm going to have a treat!" make an active choice to focus on the benefits of maintaining your Plan of Action. Let yourself hear whatever voices inside of you are suggesting that you abandon or sabotage your Lean for Life program, and pause long enough to acknowledge and respond to those voices. Encourage yourself as you would a close friend.

OLD WAY	Food thought or craving ➡	Give in ➡	Eat ➡	Feel guilty ➡	Give up
NEW WAY	Food thought or craving ➡	STOP! ➡	Take a deep breath ➡	Observe ➡	Plan of Action

The more often you do this, the more easily and effectively you'll be able to do it. That's because after you do something successfully again and again, it starts becoming spontaneous and natural. It becomes part of you. It becomes a habit.

ANY QUESTIONS?

Q: *Can I use one of the Lean for Life protein products instead of a meal?*

A: It's fine to use the protein products occasionally in place of lean meats, fish, and other food choices from your Protein list. When you do, count it as your protein serving. For long-term success, however, it's important for you to learn how to plan, shop for, and prepare appropriate meals.

Q: *Do I really need to take vitamins every day?*

A: Yes! The vitamin and mineral supplements help ensure that your body is getting the nutrients it needs—and that you'll continue feeling and looking healthy!

Q: *Can I substitute certain foods on the menu with foods that have the same number of calories?*

A: We don't recommend it. Substituting foods may change the nutritional balance of the menu, trigger hunger and cravings, and interfere with ketosis and weight loss. If it's necessary, however, be sure the food you substitute is from the same food category and contains the same amount of protein, carbohydrates, fat and calories.

Q: *Refresh my memory! What are the major benefits of staying in ketosis?*

A: When you're in mild to moderate ketosis, you'll lose weight rapidly and safely. You'll feel less hungry, less often. Your cravings will diminish. You'll have more energy and a greater sense of well-being. Most important, you'll burn excess body fat as rapidly as possible, while maintaining lean muscle mass.

Q: *Is it okay to have an extra protein snack if I'm hungry?*

A: Yes. Some individuals need more than three protein snacks a day, especially if they are active. Always carry a snack with you in case of "emergency". Remember to record your snacks and the carbohydrates on your Daily Action Plan.

DAY
5

CRAVINGS CAUSED BY PEOPLE, PLACES, EMOTIONS AND EVENTS

You can learn to change the way you respond to the forces and factors that trigger cravings.

How many times have you gone to the movies and suddenly found yourself craving popcorn? Even if you weren't hungry, your past experiences, the unmistakable aroma, the sound of kernels popping, and the sight of others eating were enough to lure you toward the concession stand.

Some people call this "Pavlovian conditioning." Back in the late 19th century, Russian scientist Ivan Pavlov conducted an experiment in which he sounded a bell when giving food to his dogs. After repeating the experiment many times, Pavlov's four-legged friends began to associate eating with the sound of the bell. They would salivate every time the bell rang, even when no food was present.

Like it or not, we have more in common with Pavlov's dogs than we might like to admit. We, too, have been conditioned, both personally and by society, to respond to certain emotions, events, and people by eating.

When you have a "conditioned response," you react without thinking. While certain conditioned responses tend to be universal—eating and drinking to excess during holidays and celebrations, for example—each of us also has unique conditioned responses. If you had a grandmother who made caramel apples every Halloween, it's a safe bet you'll develop a desire for them in late October. If your mother made hot cranberry cider every time you had a ticklish throat, odds are you're going to develop a sudden appetite for that brew the next time you're feeling sick.

CHANGING HOW YOU RESPOND

It's often difficult to permanently remove or change these cues, but you can learn how to change the ways you respond to them.

The following strategies will help you:

1. *Observe your behavior.* Identifying your conditioned responses is the first step in reprogramming them. When you're at the movies, for example, and you just "have to have popcorn," recognize what's happening. Eating popcorn at the movies is a reaction, a habit, but you don't *have* to have it. When you shift your focus away from self-defeating behavior, you'll be taking a huge step toward remaining in control. Focus instead on the film you're watching and the people you're with.

2. *Get active.* Whatever you do, don't sit and brood about how intense your cravings are. There's great truth in the adage "action equals power." Shift your attention to activities other than eating. Take a walk. Go for a swim. Head for the gym. Call a friend spur-of-the-moment and go dancing. At Lindora, we call these kinds of activities "Biomodifiers™," because they can actually change your brain and body chemistry. We'll talk more about Biomodifiers on Day 9.

FOOD for Thought

"If we all did the things we are capable of doing, we would literally astonish ourselves."

—Thomas Edison

D.D.P.P.: Changing Your Behavior

Change your response by using a process for changing behavior that we refer to as D.D.P.P.

Desire: Nothing happens until we truly want it to. Develop motivational habits to psyche yourself up every day.

Decision: "Wanting" is not enough. You must decide to stay committed and make it happen.

Plan of Action: You need a specific, detailed plan for how you will guide your behavior into successful patterns. A Plan of Action allows you to maintain control when facing challenges.

Perserverance: Stay focused and committed for as long as it takes to accomplish your goal.

3. ***Consider the consequences.*** Think ahead to tomorrow. Ask yourself how you'll feel physically and mentally if you give in to your cravings today. Do you really want to "wear" that piece of chocolate cake? Are you willing to exercise more to burn all those extra calories?

4. ***Delay your gratification.*** Cravings are like gnats. Some of them will pester you for what seems like forever, but most of them can be shooed away. The next time you're overcome with a craving, make a deal with yourself. Delay your reaction for a given period of time—an hour, three hours, one day. Tell yourself that if the craving is still as strong, you'll deal with it then. More often than not, cravings diminish or even pass within an hour or two. This is one of those rare occasions when stall tactics can be productive.

5. ***Consider alternatives.*** A craving is a suggestion, not a command. Just because the notion of stuffing yourself with cherry pie crosses your mind doesn't mean you have to actually *do* it. Whenever you feel like acting impulsively, pause long enough to explore what you're really feeling and thinking. You're likely to discover alternatives that are far more nourishing.

CONTROLLING CRAVINGS: HOW TO RESPOND TO ENVIRONMENTAL CUES

Here are several steps you can take to deal more effectively with those times that spark your desire to eat:

❏ ***Control the number of times you eat every day.*** If an extra snack helps curb your appetite, build one into your Daily Action Plan. If you can structure your eating, you'll find yourself eating less and enjoying it more.

❏ ***Be sure to eat breakfast.*** Many overweight people skip breakfast and justify it as "saving calories." Those who achieve and maintain long-term weight loss almost always eat a healthy breakfast and find doing so makes it easier to control their appetite later in the day.

❏ ***Choose one or two places in your house where you will eat.*** When you snack, go to one of your eating places and eat it. If you get the urge to nibble while watching TV, wait until your program is over, then have your meal in one of your special places.

Lean *for* Life®
DAILY ACTION PLAN

Week _____ Day _____ Date _____

Time	Meal Plans	Serving Size	(grams)
_____	**Breakfast**		
	Protein		
	Fruit or Grain		
	Beverage		
_____	**Protein Snack**		
_____	**Lunch**		
	Protein		
	Vegetable		
	Lettuce		
	Fruit		
	Beverage		
	Miscellaneous		
_____	**Protein Snack**		
_____	**Dinner**		
	Protein		
	Vegetable		
	Lettuce		
	Fruit		
	Beverage		
	Miscellaneous		
_____	**Protein Snack**		
		TOTAL	

Keto Reading _____

Weight _____

Vitamins   AM   Noon   PM

Fluids _____

Activities _____
_____
_____

Pedometer Steps _____

WEEKLY BODY MEASUREMENTS

Chest _____   Hips _____

Waist _____   Thighs _____

Abdomen _____

SUCCESS LEARNING TOOLS

Read pages # _____

Audio Tapes _____

Affirmation _____
_____

Plan to Overcome Today's Obstacles:
_____
_____
_____
_____
_____

Notes:
_____
_____
_____
_____
_____

CHOOSE ONE DAY EACH WEEK AS YOUR "PROTEIN DAY."

6. ***Review your reasons for becoming lean.*** Remind yourself why you made a commitment to becoming Lean for Life. Continue reviewing the Motivator cards you prepared on Day 1. They are effective tools to help maintain your enthusiasm and deal effectively with the people, places, emotions, and events that trigger your response to eat.

7. ***If it's really an urge to chew, then do.*** The next time you experience a craving, ask yourself whether you're craving food or if what you really want is simply to chew. Often, one has little to do with the other.

   If you're feeling tense and angry, for example, you may find yourself craving crunchy foods. This "mouth hunger" can be satisfied without jeopardizing your program. Many of the Lean for Life protein bars have a firm, chewy consistency. Cut one into small pieces and eat it slowly, over a 20-minute period, drinking water between bites. This will satisfy your hunger as well as your desire to chew. Also try sugarless gum. You can chew a piece without blowing your diet!

   The cues for cravings are all around us. How you respond to them is up to you. You're a person with goals and insight. You—not the TV, not the pastry shop, not other people—can decide what, when, and how much you'll eat.

Another Lean for Life Success Story

"I know I'm really stressed whenever I crave sweets. I get that gnawing feeling that sends me searching. I remember one time I was rifling through purses I hadn't used for months, hoping to find a piece of candy. Now that I understand what's going on, I take a deep breath and ask myself, 'What is it that I really want? Will eating really make me feel better?' The urgency usually passes, and I'm fine. These days, when I have a piece of candy, it's because I've made a conscious choice to do so."

— *Cynthia*

Your Turn

Which people, places and events trigger *your* desire to eat? What foods do you find yourself craving in various situations? Examples: "When I'm busy, I crave greasy fast food, so instead I could have an 'emergency supply' of protein bars with me...""When I'm at a ballgame, I crave hot dogs and beer, so instead I could take some turkey jerky with me..."

When I:	I crave:	Instead, I could:
_____	_____	_____
_____	_____	_____
_____	_____	_____
_____	_____	_____
_____	_____	_____
_____	_____	_____
_____	_____	_____
_____	_____	_____
_____	_____	_____
_____	_____	_____

DR. STAMPER

"Your Daily Action Plan will show you how many carbohydrates you can tolerate each day without interrupting your ketosis and your continued weight loss."

ANY QUESTIONS?

Q: *What you call environmental cues have been my downfall for years. Now that I'm aware of them, I feel much more in control. Do you have any tips for maintaining that control?*

A: These success strategies will help conquer cravings caused by environmental cues:

❑ One of the best ways to break the connection between the sight of your favorite food (an external cue) and your automatic desire to eat is not to have the food around in the first place. Eliminate as many temptations as possible. Do an inventory of your kitchen. If you find foods you don't want to be eating while you're on the program, consider giving them away or throwing them out.

❑ Remove the candy jar from the coffee table. Retire the cookie jar to a storage unit or the top shelf above the refrigerator. If they're not "staring at you," you'll be less likely to react to them out of habit. Out of sight, out of mind, out of mouth!

❑ Avoid your "danger zones." You can bolster your self-control by avoiding places you know will prompt you to eat. If the candy machine in the office break room is your downfall, take your break outdoors. If your favorite fast-food restaurant lies in wait for you on your drive home, avoid the ambush by taking an alternate route.

❑ Ask your family to eat tempting food away from home rather than bringing it into the house. While they go out for an ice cream cone, treat yourself to a brisk, energizing walk or a relaxing bubble bath.

❑ Become independent and creative. Whenever you feel tempted, remember that one of the benefits of greater awareness is greater independence. Use these occasions as reminders that you're now *acting mindfully* rather than *reacting mindlessly*.

THE DENIAL TRAP

***You'll understand what a powerful force
denial can be—and how to overcome it.***

It wasn't too many years ago that my friend Mary Beth called from her car phone to let me know she was running a few minutes late for our lunch meeting. She had stopped by her favorite department store to try on a dress and was totally exasperated.

"I swear those people must be having their clothes made in Munchkinland!" she later declared as she dragged an onion ring through the mayonnaise that had dripped from her cheeseburger. "They're cutting their clothes smaller all the time. Their size 10 used to fit me like a glove. Now I can barely fit into a 14!"

Today, Mary Beth looks back on that conversation and laughs. She now jokes that she was a real "denial diva." It's a description that, unlike the dress, fit her perfectly.

Denial is an unwillingness or refusal to accept or admit life's realities. The difference between lying and denial is simple. Lying is knowingly hiding the truth from others. Denial is unknowingly hiding the truth from ourselves.

WHY DENY?

Denial protects us from a truth that may be painful. After all, as long as we're in denial, there's no problem. And if there's no problem, then there's no need to seek solutions. Until you understand what a powerful force denial can be, you're likely to find yourself doomed to play the no-win diet game, taking two steps forward and two steps back.

Most of us have developed a variety of ways to protect ourselves from the truth. So when we decide to make significant changes in the way we think and act, it's important that we also become aware of the hidden mental patterns that block our progress and keep us mired in those unproductive patterns and behaviors.

Because we're often unaware that such patterns exist, it can be a real challenge to overcome them. At Lindora, we refer to denial and other self-protective behaviors as "defensive barriers." Another defensive barrier that often gets in the way of lasting weight loss is rationalization, which we'll take a look at tomorrow.

Recognizing and disarming defensive barriers such as denial isn't easy. In fact, it's one of those classic "Catch-22" challenges: In order to address a problem, you first have to acknowledge that there *is* a problem. Yet if you're deep in denial, it's unlikely you're going to recognize or acknowledge that you are.

BREAKING THE "INSANITY CYCLE"

Do *you* ever do the same thing over and over again and expect a different result?

While even rats in a maze eventually figure out which paths are the express lanes to nowhere, people aren't always quite so quick to get the picture. That's why the Lean for Life program focuses on changing the way you *think* as much as the way you *eat*.

To make lasting changes, first you need to gain a new awareness of how you think and how that thought process may be leading you directly down a dead-end path. Once you identify and begin eliminating your defensive barriers—those subtle, subconscious self-sabotage strategies that help keep you stuck—you'll be one step closer to shedding those pounds and *keeping* them off for life.

Lean *for* Life®
DAILY ACTION PLAN

Week _____ Day _____ Date _____

Time	Meal Plans	Serving Size	(grams)
_____	**Breakfast**		
	Protein		
	Fruit or Grain		
	Beverage		
_____	**Protein Snack**		
_____	**Lunch**		
	Protein		
	Vegetable		
	Lettuce		
	Fruit		
	Beverage		
	Miscellaneous		
_____	**Protein Snack**		
_____	**Dinner**		
	Protein		
	Vegetable		
	Lettuce		
	Fruit		
	Beverage		
	Miscellaneous		
_____	**Protein Snack**		
		TOTAL	

Keto Reading _____

Weight _____

Vitamins   AM   Noon   PM

Fluids _____

Activities _____

_____

_____

_____

\# Pedometer Steps _____

WEEKLY BODY MEASUREMENTS

Chest _____   Hips _____

Waist _____   Thighs _____

Abdomen _____

SUCCESS LEARNING TOOLS

Read pages # _____

Audio Tapes _____

Affirmation _____

_____

Plan to Overcome Today's Obstacles:

_____

_____

_____

_____

_____

Notes:

_____

_____

_____

_____

_____

_____

_____

CHOOSE ONE DAY EACH WEEK AS YOUR "PROTEIN DAY."

DISARMING DENIAL

Many people are convinced they don't have any real power over their lives. What they don't realize is that by making conscious changes in the way they *think*, they can change the way they *live*.

Making a conscious decision to break the cycle is the first step toward achieving your goal. If you want different results, you must start doing things differently. The first step is becoming more fully aware of your power to recognize and dismantle your defensive barriers and change the way you think. Until you do, your power is nothing more than unrealized potential.

In his book *The Unfair Advantage*, psychologist Tom Miller shares an analogy of a horse and rider that beautifully illustrates the relationship that exists between the conscious and the subconscious mind.

Horses are magnificent creatures. Their intelligence, however, is limited. Once a horse becomes accustomed to turning west at the first fork in the trail, convincing it to head east can become a true battle of will. The horse, being a creature of habit, will come to a stubborn standstill right in the middle of the road rather than change its routine.

But with the right strategy and plenty of patience and determination, a skilled rider can change the horse's habits, retraining it to move with grace in whatever direction the rider chooses. Even though the horse is physically bigger, the rider is mentally stronger.

WALKING: IT BENEFITS YOUR BODY *AND* YOUR BRAIN

Did you know that taking a brisk walk can actually help you think faster? Studies by Robert Dustman, director of the Neuropsychology Research Laboratory at the Veterans Affairs Medical Center Center in Salt Lake City, Utah, show that while active, aerobically fit adults over 60 retain much of the quick-wittedness of youth, adults over 40 who *don't* exercise develop undernourished neurons in their brains and don't move electrical signals as quickly. As a result, their minds slow down!

This sneak peak at "BioModifiers"—experiences or activities that can change your brain chemistry—is just one example of how you can use the mind-body connection to your advantage. We'll talk more about "BioMod" on Day 9.

Your Turn

As you read today's feature, you may have found yourself thinking "I never do that!" Take the following quiz. Every "Yes" answer would suggest that perhaps sometimes you *do*.

1. Do you ever refuse to weigh yourself because you'd rather not know? (The "What I Don't Know Won't Hurt Me" approach doesn't help avoid pain; it only delays it.)

2. Have you ever blamed the clothes dryer for tighter-fitting clothes? (Unless everyone else in your family has the same problem, this should tell you something.)

3. Do you avoid mirrors, especially when getting out of the shower?

4. Do you ever eat junk food while alone (at home or in the car) and make a point to throw away the candy, cookie, and potato chip wrappers before anyone else sees them?

5. Have you ever blamed your weight problem on "thyroid trouble," "big bones," or a "slow metabolism," even though you've never had a medical examination that supports your theories?

6. Do you ever exaggerate how long, how often, or how hard you exercise?

7. Do you blame bloat and excess weight on "water retention" resulting from your period, getting ready to begin your period, or having just had your period? (This is an especially questionable excuse if you are male!)

WHO'S IN CHARGE HERE?

Like the rider, *you*—the aware, awake, mindful you—want to be in charge of your journey. You want to be the one who decides where you're going, which route you'll travel, and how long it will take to get there. You want to have the courage to examine your motives, understand your reactions, and learn life lessons along the way.

The Lean for Life program is about gaining mastery over yourself so that you're in control. The affirmations and other mental training techniques you'll encounter in this book are effective ways to gain that mastery. At Lindora, we call this process "thought control."

Some people react strongly to this concept. The words evoke images of manipulation, as in "I don't want anyone but me controlling my thoughts!"

That's exactly the point. True thought control is not about surrendering power to anyone. It's about claiming it for yourself. By becoming more self-aware and by consciously using the mental training strategies featured in this program, you can learn to reframe your thoughts so that they are more helpful to you. When you do this consistently, new habits will emerge. You'll have an opportunity to explore thought control in more depth on Day 10.

This program has been designed for lifelong success. If you find yourself thinking that some of the procedures or information don't apply to you (we call this the "Not Me" Syndrome) or if you begin to discount

Another Lean for Life Success Story

THEN&NOW

"Defensive barriers are like blinders. You don't see the big picture. When my defensive barriers are up, immediate gratification is all that matters. I want it and I want it now. They lull you into believing that whatever you eat today doesn't matter as long as you promise to buckle down tomorrow. But until you finally break that cycle, tomorrow never comes."

—Marcia

WHAT THELMA LEARNED

Thelma was discouraged and confused.

She had been on the program for more than a week, yet she hadn't lost a pound and wasn't in ketosis.

"Maybe my body is just different," Thelma speculated. "I don't know what could be causing this."

When Jill, one of our clinic nurses, offered to review Thelma's Daily Action Plans with her, Thelma said she wasn't "a detail person" and didn't "have time" to write down what she ate and drank every day.

While telling Jill that she had been "doing the program to the letter," Thelma poured herself a cup of coffee and added three heaping spoons of non-dairy creamer.

She must have noticed Jill's expression.

"Oh, don't worry," Thelma said. "This is the 'lite' stuff."

It didn't take Sherlock Holmes to solve this mystery. Jill pointed out that a serving size of creamer was a level teaspoon. And while the "lite" non-dairy creamer had less fat, it contained the same number of calories and double the carbohydrates! Thelma was consuming 150 extra calories and 30 extra grams of carbohydrate every day without realizing it!

The bottom line? Eliminate any mystery by using correct measurements and writing down everything you eat and drink, every day, throughout "Phase 1: Weight Loss." Your Daily Action Plan is a valuable resource that allows you to identify any errors and correct them immediately.

or ignore vital features of the program, it's a clear warning sign that your defensive barriers—rationalization and denial—are firmly in place.

Don't be surprised if you find yourself resisting change along the way. In fact, expect it. People often have a definite resistance to doing things that are different from what they've done before, even when they realize that what they've done in the past no longer works. In the coming weeks, you'll discover that it's possible to overcome the mental barriers and find a new, more rewarding path.

ANY QUESTIONS?

Q: *Can I save a fruit serving from one meal and eat it later?*

A: The Menu Plan is designed to provide the appropriate balance of calories, carbohydrate, protein, fat, and fiber for each meal and snack to help you achieve the best results. Modifying the eating plan may interfere with ketosis and weight loss, and may trigger hunger and cravings.

Q: *Why is bread limited to whole grain?*

A: Whole grain bread is more nutritious, high in fiber, more filling, and less likely to trigger cravings.

Q: *Why are some meats and fish not on the menu?*

A: They're too high in natural fat and calories.

"MR. MITO" SAYS:

"People often ask, "How often—and how long—should I walk?" Our own research shows that for inactive people, almost any addition of steps to their existing routine enhances mood, energy level, sleep, and weight loss.

Three 10-minute walks a day is a realistic initial goal for almost everyone. Since walking is one of those human activities in which more is better, aim to increase your duration and distance a little every day or every other day."

RECOGNIZING RATIONALIZATION

You'll discover the benefits of changing the way you think as well as the way you eat.

When Steve returned home from work early one afternoon to find Paula eating fast-food fried chicken, he finally understood why his wife had been struggling on her weight loss program.

As always, Paula attempted to joke her way out of the situation. When it came to creative excuses, she was in a league of her own.

"It's not what you think," she insisted as she licked her fingers. "I'm just moisturizing my skin from the inside out."

When Steve didn't even smirk, Paula got testy.

"Lighten up!" she said. "It was just two tiny pieces. And anyway, I don't look that bad for a 46-year-old woman with four kids!"

Paula's ability to rationalize is hardly unique. Our defensive barriers come to the rescue whenever we want or need to protect ourselves from unpleasant feelings, difficult situations, and painful truths. Like the quills of a porcupine, these barriers are not always raised, but they're always ready if needed. They have their purpose and they serve it well.

No one would dispute that our brains are wired to protect us from physical threats. When you're at a baseball game and a foul ball zooms in your direction, you don't *think* about how to react. You duck. When you hear a loud, sudden sound, you flinch. Your eyes snap shut at an explosion of bright light. These reactions are instinctive and involuntary.

But the subtle ways in which we protect ourselves from emotional threats are much less obvious. We often react defensively, as Paula did, whenever we sense an attack on our self-image or on our worth and value as a person. Like a flinch or a blink of the eye, these reactions aren't the result of any conscious decision. In fact, we're usually not even aware of what we're doing.

One of the most common defensive barriers is rationalization. Rationalizations are excuses our minds make to help us feel better about a situation. When we rationalize, we justify our actions without acknowledging our responsibility for what has happened.

Because rationalizations are usually plausible, we can easily fool ourselves into believing them. This dilemma presents one of the greatest challenges of behavior change: How can we break a pattern when we're not even conscious it exists?

For starters, awareness is essential. Since our defensive barriers undermine our ability to change old habits, recognizing them is a fundamental step toward lasting success. To neutralize the negative impact that denial and rationalization can have in your life, use the following success strategies:

1. *Accept that your defensive barriers exist.* It's impossible to do any weight loss program successfully without coming face-to-face with your defensive barriers. If they go unrecognized, they will prevent you from achieving your goals, and you may never know why you failed.

2. *Understand the damage defensive barriers have created for you and replace them with healthier patterns.* Look at your past weight loss experiences to become more aware of how you've used rationalizations and denial to justify overeating. Can you think of one example of each? What influence did they have on your behavior? Did they really protect you or did they harm you? Knowing what you now know, what could you have done to neutralize their power?

3. *Exercise thought control.* At Lindora, we define thought control as the process in which you consciously recognize a negative or unproductive thought and immediately replace it with a positive, productive one. If you're thinking, "I want a hot fudge sundae!" substitute that thought with a conscious statement such as "I want to be lean, and every day when I make conscious choices, I'm getting closer to my goal." The process of thought control reminds you that your actions have consequences.

By exercising thought control often enough, you can change your thoughts and feelings into patterns that will help rather than hinder you. Remember that inner voice we talked about on Day 2? As you become more skilled at thought control, it will become your cheerleader. Rather than urging you to have "just one piece," it can be trained to raise the red flag and ask "What are you doing?" Carefully consider what you really want before making a decision. Ask yourself: "Is eating this now going to get me what I want and need?"

4. ***Understand that disarming defensive barriers is a process.*** Even after you fully understand how rationalizations and denial get in your way, there are still going to be times when your resistance may be down and they'll get the best of you. When this happens, acknowledge that you've slipped, learn what you can from the experience, and accept that you made a choice that you wouldn't necessarily make again. Sometimes, the lessons we learn from our mistakes are well worth the price we pay.

5. ***Remember that there may be a part of you that still resists change.*** The familiar is comforting even when it is self-defeating. It can be challenging to do things differently, even when we realize that what we've done in the past doesn't work.

6. ***Be conscious of the "Not Me" Syndrome.*** As you proceed with your program, pay careful attention to your thoughts and actions. Instead of saying "I never do that!" and discounting the advice, try following it. You may find that your defensive barriers have been keeping you away from the truth.

YOUR WEEKLY PROTEIN DAY

Beginning with your second week of Weight Loss and continuing throughout your Lean for Life program, you'll choose one day each week as your Protein Day. Follow the guidelines on pages 40-41.

"WHAT IF MY KETOSTICK IS NEGATIVE?"

You'll be checking your ketostick for color every day during "Phase 1: Weight Loss." If your stick doesn't show pink to purple color, immediately follow the guidelines on pages 41-43 to get back into ketosis as quickly as possible. As soon as you're in ketosis again, resume the Weight Loss nutritional menu.

SOUND FAMILIAR?

To appreciate how often rationalizations creep into our everyday lives, review the following and check off any of those you can remember using:

- ❏ "I deserve this. I've been good all day!"
- ❏ "Oh, it's just a little bite."
- ❏ "There are starving children in (fill in name of country)."
- ❏ "It's a shame to waste food."
- ❏ "It's Friday night."
- ❏ "It's Saturday."
- ❏ "It's Sunday."
- ❏ "It's my birthday."
- ❏ "It's fat-free."
- ❏ "I'm on vacation."
- ❏ "I paid for it, I'm eating it."
- ❏ "I'm not feeling well. I've got to eat."
- ❏ "This diet isn't good for me."
- ❏ "If I don't eat I'm going to waste away to nothing!"
- ❏ "I don't know how to make healthy foods."
- ❏ "My friend eats this and doesn't gain weight."
- ❏ "I look pretty good for my age."
- ❏ "It's a holiday."
- ❏ "It would be rude not to eat it after she made it especially for me."
- ❏ "It's no big deal."
- ❏ "I didn't eat breakfast."
- ❏ "I'll make up for it tomorrow at the gym."

How good does a rationalization have to be to work? Only good enough to lull you into temptation or to let you off the hook. Any excuse is good enough when you're looking for a reason to eat.

Lean *for* Life®
DAILY ACTION PLAN

Week _____ Day _____ Date _____

Time	Meal Plans	Serving Size	(grams)
_____	**Breakfast**		
	Protein		
	Fruit or Grain		
	Beverage		
_____	**Protein Snack**		
_____	**Lunch**		
	Protein		
	Vegetable		
	Lettuce		
	Fruit		
	Beverage		
	Miscellaneous		
_____	**Protein Snack**		
_____	**Dinner**		
	Protein		
	Vegetable		
	Lettuce		
	Fruit		
	Beverage		
	Miscellaneous		
_____	**Protein Snack**		
		TOTAL	

Keto Reading _____
Weight _____
Vitamins   AM   Noon   PM
Fluids _____

Activities
_____
_____
_____

Pedometer Steps _____

WEEKLY BODY MEASUREMENTS

Chest _____ Hips _____
Waist _____ Thighs _____
Abdomen _____

SUCCESS LEARNING TOOLS

Read pages # _____
Audio Tapes _____
Affirmation _____
_____

Plan to Overcome Today's Obstacles:
_____
_____
_____
_____
_____
_____

Notes:
_____
_____
_____
_____
_____
_____

CHOOSE ONE DAY EACH WEEK AS YOUR "PROTEIN DAY."

HOW ARE YOU DOING?

So how do you feel about your experience on the program after the first week?

Take some time to review the past week's Daily Action Plans. Are there any changes you want to incorporate in your program as you move into Week 2? More activity? Fewer snacks? More fluids? Less rationalization?

Jot down the changes and improvements you can make to enhance your results in the coming weeks.

_____

_____

_____

_____

_____

_____

_____

_____

The fine tuning you do now can have an impact on your results later!

THE MORE ENTHUSED, THE MORE YOU LOSE

You'll learn how your level of interest and enthusiasm directly impacts your degree of success.

Setting a goal is the easy part. Just ask anyone who's ever made a New Year's resolution. You begin with determination and a dream—to pay off your credit cards, to write the great American novel, to travel, to lose weight. You know what you want and vow that this time, you'll make it happen. And for a while, you do what it takes.

But then something happens. Your enthusiasm ebbs. Your focus becomes fuzzy and your determination dims. You don't give up, but you find yourself giving in. Excuses that would have never worked a week earlier are suddenly good enough. Today becomes tomorrow, and before you know it, you're back where you started, only more discouraged than before.

Sound familiar? We've all been there. Change is never easy. Consistent effort over an extended period of time isn't easy, either. If it were, we could erase the word "challenge" from the dictionary. But change *is* possible. Just ask any of the people whose inspiring success stories are included in this book. Every one of them knows an important secret: your level of interest and enthusiasm directly impacts your success. In other words, the more enthused, the more you'll lose. The more motivated you are, the more likely you will be to achieve your goal.

The challenge, of course, is maintaining your motivation over the long haul. To fully appreciate just how true this is, ask yourself the following questions:

❏ What was my goal on my last diet?

❏ Did I achieve the goal? How close did I come?

❏ How long did my enthusiasm last before I began making excuses and altering my program?

❏ How long did I maintain the weight loss I achieved?

On this program—as in life—your continued level of motivation is an important contributor to your success. It's rarely the most talented or even the luckiest person who succeeds. More often than not, those who win in life are those who stay committed and focused on the goal while others get sidetracked. Winners understand one of the basic rules of life: You can't win if you don't play the game.

JOE KNOWS

Football quarterback Joe Montana not only showed up, but consistently demonstrated the drive that made him one of sport's most respected and successful players. While some athletes struggle to maintain their focus and purpose after achieving a career pinnacle like the Super Bowl, Montana's interest and enthusiasm never wavered.

"I felt I had to prove myself every day, every game, every season," Montana said. "When I got to Notre Dame, nothing I had done at Ringgold High in Monongahela, Pennsylvania mattered. When I got to the 49'ers, nothing I had done at Notre Dame mattered. And when I got to Kansas City, nothing I had done in San Francisco mattered."

MOTIVATION MATTERS

In a *USA Today* survey, 805 American adults were asked, "What caused you to stop dieting before losing all the weight you wanted?" The top two reasons? 39% said they got "discouraged"; 24% cited a "lack of interest."

Remember: The more enthused, the more you lose!

Lean *for* Life®
DAILY ACTION PLAN

Week _____ Day _____ Date _____

Time	Meal Plans	Serving Size	(grams)
_____	**Breakfast**		
	Protein		
	Fruit or Grain		
	Beverage		
_____	**Protein Snack**		
_____	**Lunch**		
	Protein		
	Vegetable		
	Lettuce		
	Fruit		
	Beverage		
	Miscellaneous		
_____	**Protein Snack**		
_____	**Dinner**		
	Protein		
	Vegetable		
	Lettuce		
	Fruit		
	Beverage		
	Miscellaneous		
_____	**Protein Snack**		
		TOTAL	

Keto Reading _____
Weight _____
Vitamins   AM   Noon   PM
Fluids _____

Activities _____
_____
_____

Pedometer Steps _____

WEEKLY BODY MEASUREMENTS

Chest _____   Hips _____
Waist _____   Thighs _____
Abdomen _____

SUCCESS LEARNING TOOLS

Read pages # _____
Audio Tapes _____
Affirmation _____
_____

Plan to Overcome Today's Obstacles:
_____
_____
_____
_____
_____
_____
_____

Notes:
_____
_____
_____
_____
_____
_____

CHOOSE ONE DAY EACH WEEK AS YOUR "PROTEIN DAY."

DR. STAMPER

"Motivation is a decision. Remind yourself several times every day why you've decided to become Lean for Life."

Long after Montana had anything to prove to his team, his fans, or himself, he continued to demonstrate remarkable motivation and commitment. He was, above all else, consistent.

It's not enough to be interested and enthusiastic about your program *part of the time*. As you begin your second week of "Phase 1: Weight Loss," remember that *consistency counts*.

HEMINGWAY'S CONSISTENT WAYS

After interviewing writer Ernest Hemingway for *The Paris Review* in 1958, George Plimpton noted: "He keeps track of his daily progress—'so as not to kid myself'—on a large chart made out of the side of a cardboard packing case and set up against the wall under the nose of a mounted gazelle head. The numbers on the chart showing the daily output of words differ from 450, 575, 462, 1250, back to 512, the higher figures on days Hemingway puts in extra work so he won't feel guilty spending the following days fishing on the Gulf Stream."

Though Hemingway wrote nine novels and nearly 70 short stories, he was not a prolific writer. He was, however, disciplined and consistent, producing an average of two pages a day. His strategy: "Work every day. No matter what has happened the day or night before, get up and bite on the nail."

There will always be plenty of reasons why you can't, won't, or shouldn't eat well or exercise on a given day. Your challenge is to decide if you'll give those excuses enough power to derail your dream or whether you'll "bite on the nail" and stay committed enough, consistently enough, to really do it—day in and day out, no matter what.

"MR. MITO" SAYS:

"Be sure to increase your level of activity enthusiastically but gradually. If you don't increase, you won't enjoy the benefits. If you do too much too soon, you run the risk of becoming sore, fatigued, or injured. So step to it—but don't push it!"

ANY QUESTIONS?

Q: I've noticed that sometimes my breath smells and my mouth tastes bad. What's going on?

A: Ketones are excreted through the lungs as well as the kidneys. This accounts for the "keto-odor" some people occasionally notice. Make a point to brush your teeth regularly to keep your mouth fresh and clean. You might also try calorie-free breath fresheners between meals. Drinking plenty of water throughout the day will also help by keeping your mouth moist.

Q: Why can't I eat frozen diet meals from my supermarket?

A: They tend to be too low in protein and too high in calories, carbohydrates, and fat.

Your Turn

Ten days ago, you listed your reasons for becoming Lean for Life on notecards. Take a minute to review your list. Choose any one of your reasons and declare it again in writing:

"I'm learning to become Lean for Life because_____

_____

_____

_____."

After you write it down, read it out loud. This may feel a little silly at first, but revisiting your reasons is an effective way to reinforce your enthusiasm, confidence, and optimism.

Each day is a new beginning. You have good reasons to drop bad habits and stay focused on what really matters to you. This exercise is a way to start each day by celebrating your decision!

DAY
9

BIOMODIFIERS™

You can do things that will make it easier for your body to lose weight.

You've already taken two vital steps toward losing weight. You're eating foods that are high in protein and low in fat, calories, and carbohydrates. You're also exercising moderately. And it's working. In just nine days, you're already seeing and feeling results.

You're also making progress in other ways that are much less obvious. Right this minute—as you read this page—your body and mind are working together to regulate your body and create your mental state. What we've learned from our patients, and what researchers are beginning to more fully understand, is that any given task is easier to perform when you are in a particular mental state appropriate to that task.

Like most people, you probably learn best when you're relaxed and alert. But let's say you're in a situation where you need to learn something new but you're tense and tired. What can you do about it? You can change your sluggish, grumpy mental state into a relaxed, alert mental state *on purpose*. You may already be familiar with the concept of behavior modification, also known as Behavior Mod—learning to replace non-productive behaviors with behaviors that help you achieve the results you desire, such as a better job, a happier child, or a leaner, healthier body.

At Lindora, we teach a concept we call *BioModification,*™ also known as *BioMod.*™ With BioMod, you can learn to change your biochemistry and therefore your mental state from one that is *less* productive to one that is *more* productive. That's right! You can learn how to modify your mental state at will. We call this activity or experience a *BioModifier.*

People have much greater control over their mental states than previously believed. At Lindora, we had an inkling this was true in the early days when we installed "skinny mirrors" in our clinics as a way of helping patients appreciate the fact that a thinner, healthier body was possible. When patients looked into the mirrors and saw a thinner version of themselves, it helped their brains become more comfortable with the change even before it became a reality.

For many years, Dr. Stamper has also encouraged patients to cultivate what he calls an "inner smile." He counsels people who are experiencing frustration on the program to pause, take a deep breath, hold it briefly, and then visualize an internal smile as they exhale. Our patients who regularly do this report an immediate change in attitude.

Over the years, our understanding of the mind-body connection has deepened. It's clearer than ever that you can intentionally affect your mind and emotions. Through your actions you can create conditions that change your brain chemistry, and therefore change your mental state, in ways that make it easier for you to accomplish a specific purpose, such as achieving and maintaining lean weight.

A BioModifier is an experience or activity that changes what's going on in your brain. Sometimes what goes on in your brain primarily affects your mental state, and sometimes what goes on in your brain primarily affects your physical body. Sleeping, exercising, sitting in the sunshine, listening to music—these are all physical BioModifiers. Mental training techniques such as positive affirmations, mental rehearsal, and brief visualizations are mental BioModifiers.

You've already begun using a number of BioModifiers. Ketosis and exercise are examples of physical BioModifiers. By being in ketosis, for example, you're directing your brain to signal the body to increase its fat-burning capacity. By regularly engaging in moderate exercise, you stimulate your brain's ability to produce "feel-good" chemicals such as endorphins (at Lindora we call them "Lindorphins") and signal your muscle cells to make structural changes that increase fat-burning and carbohydrate metabolism.

You may also recognize that you're learning to use a number of mental BioModifiers. You're learning how to replace negative self-talk

"Success is living the life you want."

— Christopher Morley

Lean *for* Life®
DAILY ACTION PLAN

Week _____   Day _____   Date _____

Time	Meal Plans	Serving Size	(grams)
_____	**Breakfast**		
	Protein		
	Fruit or Grain		
	Beverage		
_____	**Protein Snack**		
_____	**Lunch**		
	Protein		
	Vegetable		
	Lettuce		
	Fruit		
	Beverage		
	Miscellaneous		
_____	**Protein Snack**		
_____	**Dinner**		
	Protein		
	Vegetable		
	Lettuce		
	Fruit		
	Beverage		
	Miscellaneous		
_____	**Protein Snack**		
	TOTAL		

Keto Reading _____

Weight _____

Vitamins   AM   Noon   PM

Fluids _____

Activities _____
_____
_____

Pedometer Steps _____

WEEKLY BODY MEASUREMENTS

Chest _____   Hips _____

Waist _____   Thighs _____

Abdomen _____

SUCCESS LEARNING TOOLS

Read pages # _____

Audio Tapes _____

Affirmation _____

Plan to Overcome Today's Obstacles: _____
_____
_____
_____
_____
_____

Notes: _____
_____
_____
_____
_____
_____
_____

CHOOSE ONE DAY EACH WEEK AS YOUR "PROTEIN DAY."

with positive images and messages that you are putting in place on purpose. In the days ahead you'll be learning how to use additional BioModifiers to increase your range of options.

Your mind and body are already on your side. They're working hard to help. Once you begin regularly relying on BioModifiers, it will become even easier to achieve your goal.

Your Turn

BioModifiers are things we do to help ourselves get what we want by changing what's happening in our brains and in our bodies.

What would happen if you were to give yourself permission to spend five minutes doing any of the following BioModifiers?

❏ Touch, love, and talk to your dog or cat.

❏ Take a five-minute nap.

❏ Daydream in a safe, loving place where you're completely at peace.

❏ Polish a ring or a piece of silver that has value to you.

❏ Read your favorite poem and allow yourself to absorb its form and meaning.

❏ Laugh! Call your funniest friend for a chat. Flip on the TV and watch a few minutes of your favorite old sit-coms.

❏ Enjoy looking at photographs of people you love.

❏ Put on some music and dance.

Does it work? Why not try it and find out?

WHAT DOROTHY KNOWS

Upon entering our clinics, visitors pass a wall plaque that reads "Lindora Medical Clinics: Comprehensive Weight Control." We've always thought that was a perfect description of the work we do. But if Dorothy, a 48-year-old university administrator from Los Angeles, had her way, the signs would read "Comprehensive *Life* Control."

I met Dorothy one afternoon while visiting our Westwood clinic, just a short walk from Dorothy's office on the UCLA campus. She had lost 45 pounds on the program three years earlier and had regained 10 of them over the previous six months. During that period, she explained, her life had become chaotic. She ended a long-term relationship, moved into a new home, and had been under enormous pressure at work.

"The real reason I decided to do the program again wasn't to lose the 10 pounds as much as it was to regain a sense of balance and control in my life," Dorothy explained. " When I did it the first time, I felt an incredible sense of power and purpose that spilled over into everything I did. I cultivated what I call 'life skills.' When I realized some of those skills were becoming rusty, I knew it was time for a tune-up."

Our conversation made my day. Dorothy is one of those people I think of as "daily heroes." She identified a problem, rallied her resources, and developed a plan of action. She went for it. Rather than perceiving her weight gain as a catastrophe, she chose to view it as a "wake-up call," an opportunity to refine her skills and get back in control.

When I talked with the manager of our Westwood clinic several weeks later, she mentioned that Dorothy had succeeded in losing the 10 pounds she'd regained.

I wasn't a bit surprised.

YOU ARE WHAT YOU THINK

You can learn to use your thoughts and feelings to achieve what you want.

"**W**hy do I even try? Every time I lose weight, I gain it back—and then some."

"This one piece won't hurt. And besides, who will know?"

"If I lose too much weight, I'm going to have to buy new clothes. I don't have the money or the time to shop."

"My whole family is fat. What makes me think I can be different?"

Negative thoughts like these seriously undermine your efforts to lose weight. That's why we say that to change your body, you have to change your mind.

Each of us responds to events in our lives according to how we understand and interpret what is happening to us. If our brain tells us something is dangerous, we respond one way. When it tells us something is difficult, we respond in another. And if our brain says, "This is a worthwhile challenge and you can succeed," our response is quite different.

Let's say you're meeting a friend for lunch at an Italian restaurant known for its three-cheese manicotti. You plan to order broiled fish and steamed vegetables. If you say to yourself, "I feel good about this plan.

DR. STAMPER

"Make sure you take at least 20 minutes to eat a meal. It takes that long for your stomach to tell your brain it's full."

The food will be delicious and I'll feel satisfied. I know I can do this," chances are you'll be right. You *will* be able to do it and you *will* feel good about it.

On the other hand, let's say you're feeling sorry for yourself. If you're thinking: "Why do I always have to suffer? I don't get to eat out that often. I don't think I'll be able to do it. My willpower is shot," it's a safe bet you *won't* be able to do it and you *won't* feel good about it.

Call it the power of expectation. If you expect the worst, you're more likely to get it. If self-defeating thoughts are swirling around in your head, the results you'll get are likely to be negative. The goal, of course, is to change the outcome by changing the way you react in such situations. How you *choose* to experience an event, person, place, or circumstance affects how you experience it.

If you find that negative thoughts sometimes get in your way, these success strategies can help:

1. *Listen to yourself.* Become more sensitive to your thoughts and feelings. Realize which negative messages get triggered and under what circumstances. To be successful, you need to develop different habits and skills. One of the most important is self-awareness.

2. *Replace negative thoughts and statements with positive ones.* As soon as you hear a harmful, negative message, pause and replace it with a positive one. This may sound contrived at first, but it begins to feel natural the more you do it.

   Does this mean that you tell yourself you look forward to exercise when you don't? Absolutely! You can say something like, "I love the way my body and muscles feel after I exercise. I sleep better at night and have more energy during the day." Whatever words you choose, you can counter the negative with something positive right on the spot.

   Maria, who is 18 pounds away from her weight loss goal of 86 pounds, refers to her trips to the gym as "traveling." When friends invite her to dinner, she says, "Sorry, can't tonight. I'm traveling to Italy." She loves saying it—and it reminds her of the reward she's promised herself once she achieves her goal.

3. *Practice.* Successful weight loss involves *consistently* replacing negative old patterns with positive new ones. To truly break old habits, it's important to practice the new ones again and again. "Once in a while" or "every now and then" won't cut it.

   Mental training techniques, which we'll discuss in more detail on Day 16, provide an opportunity to rehearse and practice positive patterns in your mind hundreds of times. This consistent repetition has a powerful influence and can lead to lasting change. Negative patterns of thought wither and stronger patterns of self-respect and self-confidence take their place.

This program is not just about how to lose weight and keep it off. One of our guiding principles is to teach you—and then remind you—that you always have *choices* and *options*. You can decide what to eat and what not to eat. And most important of all: You can decide what to think and what not to think.

The choices you make directly impact the results you get.

"Our life is what our thoughts make it."

— Marcus Aurelius

PARTY PLANNING

Life doesn't screech to a halt just because you've decided to lose weight. During the next several weeks, it's possible that you'll be attending a party, reception, or special event. They can be fun, but they can also be a minefield of temptation. One way to maintain your motivation is to plan ahead. These tips will help:

❑ **Nix the alcohol.** Alcohol packs a wicked triple punch. It contains empty calories. It impairs judgment and lowers your resistance to impulse eating. Alcohol also interferes with your body's ability to burn stored fat for fuel. Stick with caffeine-free diet soda or mineral water with a slice of lemon or lime.

❑ **Steer clear of buffets and party platters.** Out of sight doesn't necessarily mean out of mind, but it's a lot easier to resist that homemade potato salad or those gourmet cookies when they're on the other side of the room.

❑ **Eat before you go.** You'll find it easier to resist temptation if you're full.

❑ **Be up front.** If you're invited to a dinner party and know the host or hostess well, explain in advance that you're on the program. Ask what is being served or offer to bring something you know you can eat. You're likely to find that your host will be supportive and willing to accommodate you.

❑ **Pack protein.** Take a couple of protein snacks with you so that you always have options.

Remember: Being a guest at a party, reception, or event isn't about food—it's about good times, good conversation, and good friends.

Lean *for* Life®
DAILY ACTION PLAN

Week _____ Day _____ Date _____

Time	Meal Plans	Serving Size	(grams)
_____	**Breakfast**		
	Protein		
	Fruit or Grain		
	Beverage		
_____	**Protein Snack**		
_____	**Lunch**		
	Protein		
	Vegetable		
	Lettuce		
	Fruit		
	Beverage		
	Miscellaneous		
_____	**Protein Snack**		
_____	**Dinner**		
	Protein		
	Vegetable		
	Lettuce		
	Fruit		
	Beverage		
	Miscellaneous		
_____	**Protein Snack**		
		TOTAL	

Keto Reading _____
Weight _____
Vitamins   AM   Noon   PM
Fluids _____

Activities _____
_____
_____

Pedometer Steps _____

WEEKLY BODY MEASUREMENTS

Chest _____   Hips _____
Waist _____   Thighs _____
Abdomen _____

SUCCESS LEARNING TOOLS

Read pages # _____
Audio Tapes _____
Affirmation _____
_____
_____

Plan to Overcome Today's Obstacles:
_____
_____
_____
_____
_____
_____

Notes: _____
_____
_____
_____
_____
_____
_____
_____

CHOOSE ONE DAY EACH WEEK AS YOUR "PROTEIN DAY."

AFFIRMING THE POSITIVE

Over the next 10 days, you'll have a unique opportunity to use, think about, and react to *affirmations*. Affirmations are a form of mental rehearsal that can help you set goals, make choices, and implement new patterns of thinking and behaving.

On Day 20, we'll take a closer look at how affirmations work as BioModifiers, why they're effective, and how you can benefit from using them. Between now and then, make a point of reading the affirmations featured each day. Write them down every day on your Daily Action Plan. Say them out loud. Repeat them. Think about them. Notice your reactions.

Today's affirmation:

"I am enjoying reminding myself that I am worthy of love and respect."

DAY
11

LEARN TO MANAGE STRESS AND YOU'LL LEARN TO MANAGE FOOD

You can learn healthy new ways to manage your stress and anxiety.

Stress and food. In the grand scheme of great combinations, they rank right up there with Lucy and Ricky or fireworks and the Fourth of July. If you consider how *often* and how *automatically* we rely on food to manage our anxiety, medicate our feelings, and manipulate our moods, the link between the two is undeniable.

We've grown up in a culture in which food is much more than a source of fuel. It symbolizes a spectrum of human needs and wants, including comfort, companionship, reward, punishment, escape, control, and power.

As infants, we had bottles shoved in our mouths to relax and quiet us. As kids, we were rewarded for good behavior with cookies and candy. A friend of mine, now 41, still remembers being bribed into behaving during his dental check-ups. Twice a year, his payoff for enduring the drill without a tantrum was a hot fudge sundae on the trip home.

Food—and the withholding of it—has long been used to control children's behavior. Remember the threat of all threats: being sent to bed without supper? Even Beaver Cleaver heard that one. And how many

Lean for Life®
DAILY ACTION PLAN

Week _____ Day _____ Date _____

Time	Meal Plans	Serving Size	(grams)
_____	**Breakfast**		
	Protein		
	Fruit or Grain		
	Beverage		
	_____		
	_____		
_____	**Protein Snack**		
	_____		
_____	**Lunch**		
	Protein		
	Vegetable		
	Lettuce		
	Fruit		
	Beverage		
	Miscellaneous		
_____	**Protein Snack**		
	_____		
_____	**Dinner**		
	Protein		
	Vegetable		
	Lettuce		
	Fruit		
	Beverage		
	Miscellaneous		
	_____		
	_____		
_____	**Protein Snack**		
	_____		
		TOTAL	

Keto Reading _____
Weight _____
Vitamins   AM   Noon   PM
Fluids _____

Activities
_____
_____
_____

Pedometer Steps _____

WEEKLY BODY MEASUREMENTS

Chest _____   Hips _____
Waist _____   Thighs _____
Abdomen _____

SUCCESS LEARNING TOOLS

Read pages # _____
Audio Tapes _____
Affirmation _____
_____

Plan to Overcome Today's Obstacles: _____
_____
_____
_____
_____
_____
_____

Notes: _____
_____
_____
_____
_____
_____
_____
_____

CHOOSE ONE DAY EACH WEEK AS YOUR "PROTEIN DAY."

times was dessert the reward for cleaning your plate, even if it meant eating more than you wanted or needed?

When you look at how we've been culturally conditioned to think about and use food, it's no surprise so many of us have grown up relying on it to cope with the stress and anxiety of our everyday lives.

There are, however, a number of healthier, more effective ways to address stress. Throughout this book, you'll find suggestions for effective problem-solving strategies, mental training, and breathing exercises. Let's take a look at one of the most effective stress-reducers you can treat yourself to. It's fast, free, and easy to do. What's more, it feels terrific and offers lasting benefits.

When you're "stressed out," where do you typically feel the tension first? For most of us, stiffness and tenderness in the neck and shoulders are dead giveaways that all is not well. Rather than medicate or mask the tension by crunching potato chips or chewing cookies, try a more active, hands-on approach.

Begin by reaching up with both hands to the base of your skull, one hand under each ear. Feel the muscles and the bones. (It's only fair to warn you up front—if you're doing it correctly, it's going to be uncomfortable at first.) Press firmly against the bone without loosening the pressure and move your hands gently back and forth so that you cover the entire width and length of the muscle. Hold this as tightly as

Another Lean for Life Success Story

"I spent the first 32 years of my life using food to numb my feelings and manage my stress. I grew up in a home where sweets were my mother's solution to every problem. When I was 14, a kid I had a crush on invited my best friend to the Halloween dance. That night, my mother made me a pineapple upside-down cake. I ate the whole thing. It wasn't until I started the program that I realized how a pattern established years ago was still taking its toll. Now, rather than reaching for food whenever I'm stressed, I stop and ask myself, 'What do I really want? What do I really need?'"

—*Jessica*

you can, reminding yourself that while any discomfort you may experience is temporary, the results will be long lasting.

When you first begin doing this, make a point to apply at least one minute of uninterrupted pressure. It takes that long to begin relaxing muscle tension. After a minute or so, the pain will begin to lessen and you'll know you're doing it correctly. Continue rubbing for at least another two to four minutes.

The more you rub, the less it will hurt. Rub from the base of your skull under your ears, down the sides of your neck, and out to your shoulder blades. Repeat this several times a day to prevent the tension from recurring.

The second day you do this, expect your neck and shoulders to be tender. They may even feel bruised. Whatever you do, don't let this slow you down. This is a natural result of having worked acidic muscles so vigorously the day before. If you allow too much time to pass between rubdowns, the neck and shoulder muscles will tighten back up and you'll have to start all over again. Begin gently until it starts feeling more comfortable, than do it as vigorously as you can.

Continue this process daily. Within four to seven days, you'll find that your neck and shoulder muscles are much less tense. You'll want to give yourself a quick check-up a couple of times a week. Reach beneath the base of the skull and about the middle of the neck and press firmly. If you don't experience any significant tenderness, your neck and shoulders are tension free. If you do locate a trigger point that hurts—and sooner or later, you're bound to—massage it away.

This active approach eases away stress symptoms. Give it a chance to work for you. It's a perfect example of how your health—and your ability to enhance it—is truly in your hands.

AFFIRMATIONS

"I feel good about choosing foods that nourish me and keep me healthy."

"KETO-CONSISTENCY" COUNTS

Consistency is one of the "secrets" of success on this program. Once you're in ketosis, stay there. Why make Weight Loss more challenging than it needs to be? If you discover you're not in ketosis, review your previous day's Action Plan to see where the excess carbohydrates came from. Then take action and follow the guidelines on pages 41-43.

Your Turn

What causes you stress? By identifying the people, places, events, and circumstances that cause stress in your life, you will become more aware of how your stress can influence *what* you eat, *when* you eat, and *how often* you eat.

Put a mark next to the statements that you generally find to be true:

❏   My work is too demanding.

❏   I don't like my job.

❏   My family responsibilities often feel overwhelming.

❏   I'm self-conscious about my appearance and/or concerned about my weight.

❏   I don't have enough fun or "down time" to do what I want.

❏   I worry about my personal safety.

❏   I've been divorced or separated within the last year.

❏   Someone I care about has been ill or has died within the last year.

❏   I'm concerned about my job security.

❏   I worry about my health.

❏   I have difficulty communicating with my boss and/or co-workers.

❏   I'm fighting regularly with a relative or friend.

❏   My income is too low to meet my monthly bills.

❏   I became a parent within the last year.

❏   I am a care-giver to a family member or friend.

❏   I recently made a large purchase (house, car, tuition).

❏   I've moved within the last year.

❏   I'm concerned about my level of physical fitness.

List any other ongoing or major causes of stress in your life:

_____

_____

_____

HOW DO YOU REACT–AND RESPOND–TO STRESS?

Now that you've identified your major sources of stress, let's look at how you respond. What impact does stress have on your body, your brain, and your behavior? Review the following list. Circle 0 for never, 1 for sometimes, and 2 for always.

I notice the following physical responses to stress:

0	1	2	headaches
0	1	2	change in attitude
0	1	2	fatigue
0	1	2	interrupted sleep/sleeping too much
0	1	2	indigestion
0	1	2	sore back and/or shoulder muscles

In my behavior, I notice:

0	1	2	decreased productivity
0	1	2	increased irritability and anger
0	1	2	increased eating and snacking
0	1	2	increased smoking
0	1	2	increased drug or alcohol intake
0	1	2	increased spending
0	1	2	withdrawal and a desire not to be bothered by others

I notice the following psychological responses to stress:

0	1	2	sadness or depression
0	1	2	difficulty concentrating
0	1	2	feeling emotionally drained
0	1	2	feeling impulsive
0	1	2	forgetfulness
0	1	2	a desire to eat more
0	1	2	feeling anxious or short-tempered

The more 2's you've circled, the more attention you need to pay to how you manage your stress.

Over the next several days, notice how you respond to stress. Do you eat more than you want or need? Consider how BioModifiers (review Day 9) can help change the signal you're sending your brain from "Eat!" to "Let's do something positive."

ANY QUESTIONS?

Q: *I love walking for a few minutes, but I get bored easily. Any suggestions?*

A: Do you ever use a stereo headset while walking? Time flies when you listen to talk radio, books on tape, or your favorite music. You might also invite a friend, neighbor, or family member to join you.

     Make a point to include a variety of activities in your weekly schedule. Go bicycling. Try the stair climbing, rowing, or cross-country ski machines at your gym. Dance to your favorite music—even if it's alone in your living room. Whatever you do, remember to do it *moderately*.

     These kinds of activities will help you avoid falling into a rut. They'll also reduce the risk of injury or quitting the program that

Another Lean for Life Success Story

THEN&NOW

"When I began the program, I focused on the 43 pounds I wanted to lose. It never occurred to me that what I might gain would turn out to be every bit as meaningful. The strategies and skills I learned have enhanced my health, my relationships, and my work. I no longer see my future as something that will happen to me. I now realize that the choices I make—or don't make—today directly affect the quality of my life tomorrow."

— *Laura*

WHO'S IN CHARGE OF YOUR 'INNER COMMITTEE'?

You will learn how your "inner voices" compete for your attention.

Grace is an accomplished artist. In recent years, she has earned a national reputation for her dramatic murals. Her work is featured in top galleries and her first one-woman exhibit opened to rave reviews. Yet there are days when Grace wakes up feeling like a fraud, wondering when the world will discover she has no talent.

A.J. is the most outgoing, fun-loving character in his fraternity. He's a practical joker with an offbeat sense of humor and a magnetic personality. There are days, however, when the thought of interacting with people makes A.J. cringe. He retreats to his bedroom, unplugs his phone, and listens to music for hours at a time.

Monica is ecstatic about her weight loss success. She's lost 27 pounds and is more than halfway to her goal. But there are times, she admits, when she finds herself questioning whether her goal is "really worth the effort" and whether she has "whatever it takes" to maintain her weight loss.

Like Grace, A.J., and Monica, we all experience an array of contradictory emotions that influence how we think, act, and feel. Within each of us exists an "Inner Committee" of conflicting voices

"We ask ourselves, 'who am I to be brilliant, gorgeous, talented, and fabulous?' Actually, who are you not to be?"

— Marianne Williamson

competing to be heard. One of your inner voices is loving and supportive. Another is harsh and critical. There's a frightened one, a joyful one, and an angry one. There's even a curious, playful one.

While each of these inner voices has a point of view and an agenda, you are ultimately the "chairperson" of your Inner Committee. Every thinking, responsible person has moments when "I can't" or "I won't" messages threaten to limit his or her options. By strengthening the positive inner voices that are open, loving, and supportive, you can free yourself to move forward and manage your moments of self-doubt more effectively.

Until you understand how this chorus of inner voices works, it's easy to feel confused. But once you do, you can learn to rely on your Inner Committee to help you zero in on what's really important to you.

Perhaps you can recognize some or all of these common voices, as well as adding several of your own:

Your Frightened Voice	"I'm afraid I'm not going to do this right."
Your Angry Voice	"I'm never allowed to do or say what I want!"
Your Critical Voice	"Don't even bother— you don't deserve it."
Your Joyful Voice	"Hey, let's do this! This is wonderful!"
Your Curious Voice	"I'll figure out a way to do this!"
Your Loving Voice	"I'm with you—no matter what!"
Your Confident Voice	"I can do it!"

Considering the various voices vying for power and control, it's no wonder we sometimes feel or think one thing today, only to feel or think something quite different tomorrow. Understanding these apparent contradictions can help you develop a balanced perspective on your inner conflicts. It can also remind you that whatever voice is speaking at the moment isn't the only voice with something to say.

There are times when one of your voices may sound especially shrill, obnoxious, or destructive. It's important to listen to all of them, not only those that are pleasant and encouraging. The voices that are afraid or angry often perform an important service in alerting us to be cautious.

Lean *for* Life®
DAILY ACTION PLAN

Week _____   Day _____   Date _____

Time	Meal Plans	Serving Size	(grams)
_____	**Breakfast**		
	Protein		
	Fruit or Grain		
	Beverage		
_____	**Protein Snack**		
_____	**Lunch**		
	Protein		
	Vegetable		
	Lettuce		
	Fruit		
	Beverage		
	Miscellaneous		
_____	**Protein Snack**		
_____	**Dinner**		
	Protein		
	Vegetable		
	Lettuce		
	Fruit		
	Beverage		
	Miscellaneous		
_____	**Protein Snack**		
		TOTAL	

Keto Reading _____
Weight _____
Vitamins   AM   Noon   PM
Fluids _____

Activities _____
_____
_____
_____

Pedometer Steps _____

WEEKLY BODY MEASUREMENTS

Chest _____   Hips _____
Waist _____   Thighs _____
Abdomen _____

SUCCESS LEARNING TOOLS

Read pages # _____
Audio Tapes _____
Affirmation _____
_____

Plan to Overcome Today's Obstacles:
_____
_____
_____
_____
_____
_____

Notes:
_____
_____
_____
_____

CHOOSE ONE DAY EACH WEEK AS YOUR "PROTEIN DAY."

DEALING WITH SELF-DOUBT

What do you do when you hear your Critical Voice, the one that says:

"I know myself—I'll do fine on this program for a while, then I'll put all the weight right back on."?

For starters, you want to recognize it and respond as the adult in charge, perhaps with something as simple as, "I choose to ignore what you're saying right now and continue my weight loss plans." In addition, you also want to do everything you can to strengthen the powerful, positive voice that knows you will be successful. This requires setting aside some time every day for mental training practice, just as you would for physical exercise. This needs to be protected time when you know you won't be interrupted.

You can also "sit in" on a meeting of your Inner Committee. Write down what your different voices are saying, as well as your response to them. Make note of the negative comments you're hearing, but focus primarily on what your loving, joyful, curious, confident voices say to counter negative messages. Cultivate strong positive voices so that they can overpower the negative ones.

Let's say, for example, you're beginning to notice changes in how you look and feel. While part of you will be thrilled and think, "I knew you could do it!" there may also be a part that's terrified by your progress. You may hear an antagonistic voice—perhaps a combination of your Frightened Voice ("I'm afraid I'm not going to do this right") and your Critical Voice ("Don't even bother—you don't deserve it!").

When most of us hear our negative inner voices, our first inclination is to silence or ignore them. There is, however, another possibility. Whenever you become aware of a negative voice, you can welcome the fact that you're being warned of possible self-sabotage. Listen carefully to what the voice is saying. Is it telling you something you need to hear? If it's simply afraid and reflecting old doubts, reassure it. Tell yourself it will be okay, just as you would tell a child in need of comfort. Then do what you've decided is in your best interest.

Remember: The members of your Inner Committee aren't issuing commands. They're merely voicing fears and concerns. The decision as to which voice has the greater influence is ultimately yours.

Your Turn

Since you began your program, it's a safe bet the voices that populate your Inner Committee have each had something to say. Which have the greatest power? Which seem most persistent? Write down a message that each of your inner voices has sent since you started the program.

Your Frightened Voice "_____"

Your Angry Voice "_____"

Your Critical Voice "_____"

Your Joyful Voice "_____"

Your Curious Voice "_____"

Your Loving Voice "_____"

Your Confident Voice "_____"

Another Lean for Life Success Story

"I know it sounds weird, but I visualize the Seven Dwarfs when I think of my Inner Committee. Before I started the program, Grumpy had a lot of power. So did Bashful. I always listened to the inner voice that told me not to take risks or try anything new. Now that I've lost 26 pounds, I hear a lot more from Happy. Grumpy and Bashful still try to exert their influence, but I remind myself that they only have as much power as I give them. How I choose to feel— and what I choose to do—is totally up to me."

Then & Now

— *Kyle*

AFFIRMATIONS

"I am worthy
of love
and respect."

ANY QUESTIONS?

Q: Even when I'm in ketosis, my ketostick never turns dark purple. Why not?

A: The color on your ketostick can be influenced by a number of factors. Any color from light pink to dark purple indicates you're in ketosis. Some people never have a dark purple ketostick because of individual variations in their body's physiology. If you make a diet error and eat too many carbohydrates, your body won't be burning fat, you won't be in ketosis, and you won't have color on your ketostick. On Weight Loss menu days, your ketostick will typically show a lighter color than on Protein Days because your menu includes more carbohydrates.

"MR. MITO" SAYS:

The New England Journal of Medicine *published the findings of a study involving obese subjects who reported they were unable to lose weight despite a history of strict dieting. The obese subjects described themselves as being in control of their eating behavior, and believed their obesity was due to a low metabolism and not overeating. Although the subjects believed they were accurately reporting their food intake, the results of the study showed they were actually underreporting it. In addition, they overestimated the amount of energy they expended in physical activity. In other words, they ate more and exercised less than they realized. Their inability to lose weight was concluded to be the result of a misperception of their caloric intake and energy expenditure rather than from a genetic, medical or metabolic cause.*

This study illustrates why it's important to accurately and consistently complete your Daily Action Plan and record your pedometer steps. How are you doing with yours?

TURNING OBSTACLES INTO OPPORTUNITIES

You can learn how to see problems as possibilities for personal growth—and you can become more skilled at solving them.

Amelia Earhart. Jackie Robinson. Michelangelo Buonarroti. Barbara Jordan. Dr. Jonas Salk. Helen Keller. Thomas Edison. Wolfgang Amadeus Mozart.

These extraordinary achievers have more in common than a place in the history books. Every one of them faced—and overcame—tremendous obstacles in order to make their marks in the world. Yet as unique as their gifts and achievements were, you can bet they each experienced their share of setbacks, fear, frustration, disappointment, and self-doubt.

Anyone who has ever accomplished anything has encountered challenges along the way. Writer Huston Smith, a student and teacher of the world's great religions, believes that our problems are a gift, an opportunity life offers so that we may make spiritual discoveries. In learning to overcome difficulties, Smith suggests, we learn to search for answers, to struggle with life's greater issues, and to experience growth.

While it's doubtful that most people would think of the obstacles encountered on a weight loss program as "spiritual," the character traits

"All things are difficult before they are easy."

— Thomas Fuller

we develop when we face challenges—patience, insight, vision, focus, and self-respect, among others—can bolster and strengthen our spirit and sense of mastery on this or any other self-improvement pursuit.

Over the past 12 days, it's likely that you've found yourself in situations where you didn't respond as well as you would have liked. Maybe there was a night when your cravings got the best of you. Perhaps you skipped your exercise or decided to "test" the program by seeing whether you could eat your favorite food and still remain in ketosis.

Whatever obstacles you face on this program, remember that you always have a *choice* as to how to react. You can choose to feel bad and give up, or you can use your experience as an opportunity to learn and grow. Your attitude—the mindset with which you approach problems—has a direct impact on your ability to transform obstacles into opportunities.

People who consistently demonstrate this positive "achievement attitude" share three common traits—belief, desire, and persistence:

1. ***They believe it's possible to improve their situation.*** When you believe that what you do influences the results you get, you will see yourself as someone who can act effectively to get what you want.

2. ***They have a genuine desire to improve their situation.*** Not everyone wants to improve his or her life. Sometimes we become so comfortable with our problems that they fit like an old slipper. It's hard to give them up. Problems sometimes serve a purpose, such as helping us avoid the challenge of change, or keeping others at a distance. Next time you're grappling with a problem, ask yourself how much you *really* want to solve it. Are there hidden payoffs for *not* overcoming the problem? What, if anything, are you getting out of staying "stuck"?

3. ***They are persistent in improving their situation.*** A recent article in *Parade* featured women who had beaten enormous odds to achieve greatness. All of them—the college president, the business entreprenuer, the breast-cancer researcher, the naval educator—talked about the importance of tenacity and trying a variety of approaches until one finally worked. They refused to give up. For them, failure was not an option.

As you near the halfway mark of the Weight Loss module, ask yourself: "Do I possess an 'achievement attitude?' Do I believe in my ability to accomplish my goal?"

If so, what can you do in the coming weeks to reinforce it? If not, what's stopping you right now from applying what you've learned to transform your obstacles into opportunities?

Lean *for* Life®
DAILY ACTION PLAN

Week _____ Day _____ Date _____

Time	Meal Plans	Serving Size	(grams)
_____	**Breakfast**		
	Protein		
	Fruit or Grain		
	Beverage		
_____	**Protein Snack**		
_____	**Lunch**		
	Protein		
	Vegetable		
	Lettuce		
	Fruit		
	Beverage		
	Miscellaneous		
_____	**Protein Snack**		
_____	**Dinner**		
	Protein		
	Vegetable		
	Lettuce		
	Fruit		
	Beverage		
	Miscellaneous		
_____	**Protein Snack**		
		TOTAL	

Keto Reading _____
Weight _____
Vitamins   AM   Noon   PM
Fluids _____

Activities
_____
_____
_____

Pedometer Steps _____

WEEKLY BODY MEASUREMENTS

Chest _____ Hips _____
Waist _____ Thighs _____
Abdomen _____

SUCCESS LEARNING TOOLS

Read pages # _____
Audio Tapes _____
Affirmation _____

Plan to Overcome Today's Obstacles:
_____
_____
_____
_____
_____
_____

Notes:
_____
_____
_____
_____
_____
_____
_____

CHOOSE ONE DAY EACH WEEK AS YOUR "PROTEIN DAY."

Your Turn

Write down three goals you've accomplished in the past five years that you're especially proud of:

1. _____

2. _____

3. _____

List three specific skills, abilities, attitudes, or behaviors that contributed to each of those successes:

Goal #1	Goal #2	Goal #3
_____	_____	_____
_____	_____	_____
_____	_____	_____

Review this list. Are you currently using all of the resources that have helped you succeed in the past? If your answer isn't "Yes," consider how you can more effectively support yourself in achieving your goal.

"MR. MITO" SAYS:

"Studies show that people who begin their day with a healthy breakfast are better able to control their calorie intake throughout the rest of the day. In addition to providing energy and nutrition, breakfast also helps moderate appetite, which makes it easier to avoid midday munchies and binges. Eating a healthy breakfast raises the metabolism for increased calorie burning. Breakfast also benefits your brain as well as your body: studies reveal that breakfast-eaters do better on cognitive tests than breakfast-skippers."

THE EXERCISE ADVANTAGE

Moderate exercise is an investment in your health that:

- ❏ releases tension and promotes relaxation.
- ❏ naturally controls your appetite.
- ❏ accelerates weight loss by increasing mitochondria and burning calories that would otherwise be stored as fat.
- ❏ strengthens your immune system.
- ❏ produces norepinephrine, a chemical that naturally elevates your mood and works as an antidepressant.
- ❏ enhances your overall sense of well-being.
- ❏ tones and firms muscles.
- ❏ helps boost your metabolism.
- ❏ increases your strength and stamina.
- ❏ helps you sleep better.
- ❏ improves your overall flexibility, balance, and coordination.

"I am enjoying doing the things that are helping me become lean and healthy."

DAY 14

PROBLEM SOLVING

You will discover how to solve problems and embrace challenge and change.

Ingrid and Robin are living proof that opposites sometimes attract. They've been best friends since meeting in the second grade nearly 20 years ago. But other than their childhoods and a mutual desire to drop 30 pounds before their upcoming high school reunion, they seem to have little in common.

Ingrid, who recently started her own gourmet catering business, is adventurous, animated, and single. She loves a challenge as much as life itself. Robin, a court reporter who married her college sweetheart five years ago, is much more reserved and conservative. A homebody, she values security and enjoys routine.

Even the way the two friends resolve problems and deal with conflict is as different as night and day. Ingrid considers problems to be an inevitable part of life. She sees them as temporary challenges to be overcome. "You can't have a rainbow," she's fond of saying, "if you don't have the rain."

While Ingrid has always been one to *make* things happen, Robin prefers to *let* things happen. Never one to embrace challenge or change, she procrastinates and passively avoids problems whenever possible.

Robin freely admits that if Ingrid hadn't prodded her to do the Lean for Life program with her, she probably would "never have gotten around to it."

WHAT'S YOUR PROBLEM-SOLVING STYLE?

Ingrid and Robin operate on opposite ends of the problem-solving spectrum. Most of us function somewhere in the middle. We typically welcome some challenges and handle some problems with ease and efficiency, while dodging other challenges and avoiding other problems at all costs.

One of the strongest predictors of success at any endeavor—including weight loss—is one's belief that he or she can solve problems effectively and achieve a desired result. While there's no one "right" way to solve problems or resolve conflicts, this straighforward five-step strategy can be a valuable tool for resolving whatever problems you encounter on your program—and in life:

1. ***Identify the problem.*** Sounds obvious enough, doesn't it? It is. But sometimes it's so easy to get so wrapped up in how you're reacting to a situation or circumstance that the actual reason you're feeling bad can get lost in the shuffle. Anxiety, uncertainty, anger, depression, disappointment, confusion, guilt, and feelings of inadequacy are all common responses to everyday problems. They aren't, however, the problem itself.

DR. STAMPER

"Food is the most inexpensive, readily available, socially acceptable drug in the world."

REWARD YOURSELF

One great way to stay motivated on the program is to reward yourself as you achieve intermediate goals.

Janet, who is just 12 pounds away from her 50-pound weight loss goal, treated herself to a manicure when she lost 10 pounds. After she lost 20, she went back for a facial. She celebrated the 30 pound mark by buying a bicycle. And when she celebrates her one-year anniversary, Janet and her best friend plan to celebrate with a ski trip to Lake Tahoe.

How are *you* rewarding yourself? Be sure to celebrate your success along the way. It's a terrific way to stay focused—and to recognize a job well done!

Lean *for* Life®
DAILY ACTION PLAN

Week _____   Day _____   Date _____

Time	Meal Plans	Serving Size	(grams)
_____	**Breakfast**		
	Protein		
	Fruit or Grain		
	Beverage		
_____	**Protein Snack**		
_____	**Lunch**		
	Protein		
	Vegetable		
	Lettuce		
	Fruit		
	Beverage		
	Miscellaneous		
_____	**Protein Snack**		
_____	**Dinner**		
	Protein		
	Vegetable		
	Lettuce		
	Fruit		
	Beverage		
	Miscellaneous		
_____	**Protein Snack**		
	TOTAL		

Keto Reading _____
Weight _____
Vitamins   AM   Noon   PM
Fluids _____

Activities
_____
_____
_____

Pedometer Steps _____

WEEKLY BODY MEASUREMENTS

Chest _____   Hips _____
Waist _____   Thighs _____
Abdomen _____

SUCCESS LEARNING TOOLS

Read pages # _____
Audio Tapes _____
Affirmation _____
_____

Plan to Overcome Today's Obstacles:
_____
_____
_____
_____
_____
_____

Notes:
_____
_____
_____
_____
_____
_____

CHOOSE ONE DAY EACH WEEK AS YOUR "PROTEIN DAY."

Ask yourself what's really going on. Rather than reacting or getting caught up in how you're feeling, do your best to objectively identify and define what's truly troubling you. Our patients often find it helpful to write the problem down in a clear, simple sentence. A problem well defined is a problem half solved.

2. **Create a list of possible solutions.** Brainstorm all the ways you can think of to solve the problem. As you write down all the options that come to mind, ignore your critical inner voice, the one that says things like, "That'll never work!"

3. **Choose the best solution.** In many cases, more than one solution will work, yet one is likely to emerge as more effective and productive than the others.

4. **Set realistic goals.** *You want your goals to be big enough to matter, small enough to achieve, and safe enough to tolerate.* Think of your goal as a dream with a deadline, then make it happen!

If, for example, your problem is eating too much at night, the solution you came up with may have been to eat a mid-afternoon

AFFIRMATIONS

"I like seeing myself as an effective problem solver."

Your Turn

It's been two weeks since you first took your measurements. It's time to do it again!

Measure your chest, waist, lower abdomen, hips, and upper thigh, and jot down the numbers below. This is a useful way to keep track of fat loss.

Chest _____   Hips _____

Waist _____   Thigh _____

Abdomen _____

Compare your results with your measurements from "Prep: Day 2." How many total inches have you lost? Where did you lose most?

On Day 28, you'll be comparing your measurements with today's numbers, so keep up the good work!

snack so you're not ravenous and out of control. An appropriate goal could be to pack a mid-afternoon snack every morning before leaving for work.

5. ***Follow through.*** Did you go to the grocery store to buy your snacks? Did you prepare your snack at home so you could take it with you? Did it actually make its way into your purse or briefcase? Last but not least, did you eat your mid-afternoon snack sometime mid-afternoon?

Each of these steps counts. A plan without action is just an idea. You'll find problem-solving easier when you have written down your problem, the solution you've decided to follow, the goals you've set, and the steps needed to achieve the goal.

YOUR PERSONAL SATISFACTION QUOTIENT

How you feel about your life—your work, your family, your relationships, your finances, your health, your body— impacts everything you think, say, and do. Are you physically energetic? Are you happy more often than sad? Do you get along with others? Do you like yourself? Circle the number that reflects how you feel about your life *at this moment*:

| 1 | 2 | 3 | 4 | 5 | 6 | 7 | 8 | 9 | 10 |

I've never been more unhappy.

I'm generally satisfied with my life.

My life is terrific!

You did this exercise on "Prep: Day 2." Refer back to page 56 to see whether your answer has changed. If so, what changes does today's score reflect?

VALUES AND VISION

You can create a personal vision that will guide you toward changing your life for the better.

What matters to you? What do you value? How do those values influence your vision of your future?

While these may not be questions you often ask yourself, the answers are reflected every day in the way you live. Your values—the basic principles you live by—directly affect your behavior and decisions. They also influence what you expect and what you'll accept.

What follows is a powerful exercise that has transformed lives. It can help you clarify your values and declare your vision in a way that can provide direction and purpose. The power of this exercise is that it lets you experience yourself—in your imagination—*already being the person you want to be,* having already overcome whatever obstacles await you. *You get to experience yourself already enjoying success, even before the actual changes have taken place.*

During this exercise, you're likely to discover things about yourself that your rational, logical mind might not have noticed before. It may be the first time you've ever seriously questioned what really matters to you.

"I am enjoying my
moderate exercise."

HOW TO CREATE YOUR VISION STATEMENT

To get the most out of this experience, do it when you're feeling relaxed and receptive. Set aside at least 20 minutes and choose a setting that feels comfortable.

Read the narrative in the "Your Turn" box on the following page. When you come to the passage that invites you to experience yourself saying, "This is what I have, this is what I'm doing as part of my daily life, this is who I am," close your eyes and let yourself enjoy this richly satisfying process.

Take the time to fully experience every part of this vision, adding all the sensory details you can. The more completely you enter into your vision, taking time to experience the scene and the feelings it generates, the more of a guide and an inspiration your vision will be.

THE NEXT STEP

After you've reflected on your vision, write it out in as much detail as you can. What does your life look and feel like? Who are you? How is the person in your vision different from who you are now? Who is sharing it all with you?

Once you've finished, take a few minutes to reread it and fully appreciate what you have created. It's a precious document that clarifies your goals and expectations, who you are, and what's truly important to you.

It's a roadmap to your future.

Another Lean for Life Success Story

"I just sort of took life as it came until the day I did my Vision Statement. It was a real wake-up call. It forced me to take an honest look at what I was—and wasn't—doing to create the healthy, independent lifestyle I always said I wanted. Since I completed the Lean for Life program nine months ago, I've maintained a 42-pound weight loss and enrolled in school to become a massage therapist. It's not always easy, but I have a sense of pride and purpose I never felt before. It feels terrific."

THEN&NOW

— Gwen

MY VISION STATEMENT

I am waking up in the morning... I'm excited about being alive, excited about the things I will be doing today.

At this moment, I have no need to hurry. I look out the window and see that the sky is crystal clear and beautiful.

I stretch and smile. I let myself become aware of the gifts I've been given... aware of the work I've done... of what I've accomplished... of what I have now... of what I'm doing in my daily life... of who I am. This feels exactly right! I have so much to be grateful for.

This is what I have, this is what I am doing as part of my daily life, this is who I am:

_____

_____

_____

_____

_____

_____

I feel satisfaction in knowing that I am doing what is important to me. I live with a feeling of accomplishment and with a deep sense of inner peace.

My life is full and I feel very much alive. I'm committed to continuing to do the things that help me take care of myself physically, emotionally, intellectually, spiritually, and in every other way.

I'm feeling safe, strong and comfortable. It feels good to know that I deserve all this, and that I'm doing what is important to me.

"You gain strength, courage, and confidence by every experience in which you really stop to look fear in the face. You must do the things you cannot do."

—Eleanor Roosevelt

Lean *for* Life®
DAILY ACTION PLAN

Week _____ Day _____ Date _____

Time	Meal Plans	Serving Size	(grams)
_____	**Breakfast**		
	Protein		
	Fruit or Grain		
	Beverage		
_____	**Protein Snack**		
_____	**Lunch**		
	Protein		
	Vegetable		
	Lettuce		
	Fruit		
	Beverage		
	Miscellaneous		
_____	**Protein Snack**		
_____	**Dinner**		
	Protein		
	Vegetable		
	Lettuce		
	Fruit		
	Beverage		
	Miscellaneous		
_____	**Protein Snack**		
	TOTAL		

Keto Reading _____
Weight _____
Vitamins   AM   Noon   PM
Fluids _____

Activities _____
_____
_____

Pedometer Steps _____

WEEKLY BODY MEASUREMENTS

Chest _____   Hips _____
Waist _____   Thighs _____
Abdomen _____

SUCCESS LEARNING TOOLS

Read pages # _____
Audio Tapes _____
Affirmation _____
_____
_____

Plan to Overcome Today's Obstacles:
_____
_____
_____
_____
_____

Notes: _____
_____
_____
_____
_____
_____
_____

CHOOSE ONE DAY EACH WEEK AS YOUR "PROTEIN DAY."

ANY QUESTIONS?

Q: *When shouldn't I exercise? When should I take it slow?*

A: Skip your regular exercise whenever you have a fever. (If your fever is caused by a viral infection, exercise can increase the risk of the virus causing inflammation of your heart muscle.) If you've been away from your ordinary routine for four days or more, it's a good idea to ease back into it gradually. After any injury or surgery, it's a good idea to consult with your health professional before returning to exercise.

Q: *Is it okay to skip a day if I just don't feel like exercising?*

A: Okay with whom?

DAY 16

IF YOU WANT TO CHANGE YOUR BODY, YOU HAVE TO CHANGE YOUR MIND

*You can learn to tell your brain
what to tell your body.*

I f you've ever lost weight and then regained it—as most of us have—the mental training techniques you'll be learning today may be just the "something" you need to get off the diet roller coaster once and for all.

What you think, how you feel, how you plan, and what you expect determines the decisions you make and how well you carry them out. By strengthening the connection between your body and your mind, you can enhance your success.

Here's how the nurses in our clinics explain the process:

1. *Your brain tells the rest of your body what to do.* It sends messages by way of nerve signals and chemicals released into the bloodstream. These messages influence your body's structure, functioning, and observable actions.

2. *Your brain knows what the rest of your body is doing.* The rest of your body sends messages back to the brain.

3. ***You can tell your brain what to tell your body right now.*** You can trigger short-term changes inside your body, and you can enact whatever actions you have decided to carry out.

4. ***You can post instructions inside your brain to be used later.*** Your brain is like a computer. It can be programmed to activate a certain function at a later time. You can let your brain know what messages to send to the rest of your body when you are under stress, paying attention to something else, or acting automatically, out of habit.

TELL ME MORE

Until recently, medical students were taught that the structure of the brain changed very little after childhood. Only within the past 20 years have scientists discovered that the physical connections among nerve cells in the brain evolve throughout our lives as we continue to have life experiences. These patterns determine what messages the brain sends to the body and the conditions under which those messages are sent. What's more, we now know that we can change and strengthen these patterns if we so choose.

It's exciting to be able to tap into the incredible power that exists within us. It's especially intriguing to know that power can be accessed quickly to help achieve a specific goal. I know this can happen because I've done it. During an especially demanding three-month period several years ago, I was called upon to make a major presentation at a national medical convention. I also wanted to participate in a business-related golf tournament, even though I hadn't picked up a golf club in nearly five years. These events both surfaced at a time when I was developing a long-range strategic plan for Lindora that had to be completed for a presentation.

I knew something had to give—but what? The questions were more obvious than the answers. Could I do it all? Could I do it all *well?* How would I deal with the emotional, physical, and intellectual challenges that awaited me? How could I most effectively rally my resources to achieve my goals?

Once I clarified the challenge, I was determined to find the answers. I sought out Herman M. Frankel, M.D., and Jean Staeheli of Portland Health Institute, Inc., in Portland, Oregon. I was familiar with their groundbreaking mental training work and extraordinary success with Olympic and other world-class athletes, classical musicians, corporate executives, patients facing major surgery, people with chronic illness, trial witnesses, and others confronting life crises or crossroads. I was curious whether I could effectively apply their techniques to achieve my business-related goals, as well as to my goal of quickly enhancing my golf game.

DR. STAMPER

"Train the brain and the body will follow! The mental training techniques described today are extremely powerful. When practiced consistently, they can help you enhance your performance in many areas of your life."

Lean for Life®
DAILY ACTION PLAN

Week _____ Day _____ Date _____

Time	Meal Plans	Serving Size	(grams)
_____	**Breakfast**		
	Protein		
	Fruit or Grain		
	Beverage		
_____	**Protein Snack**		
_____	**Lunch**		
	Protein		
	Vegetable		
	Lettuce		
	Fruit		
	Beverage		
	Miscellaneous		
_____	**Protein Snack**		
_____	**Dinner**		
	Protein		
	Vegetable		
	Lettuce		
	Fruit		
	Beverage		
	Miscellaneous		
_____	**Protein Snack**		
		TOTAL	

Keto Reading _____

Weight _____

Vitamins   AM   Noon   PM

Fluids _____

Activities _____
_____
_____

Pedometer Steps _____

WEEKLY BODY MEASUREMENTS

Chest _____ Hips _____

Waist _____ Thighs _____

Abdomen _____

SUCCESS LEARNING TOOLS

Read pages # _____

Audio Tapes _____

Affirmation _____
_____

Plan to Overcome Today's Obstacles:
_____
_____
_____
_____
_____
_____

Notes:
_____
_____
_____
_____
_____
_____

CHOOSE ONE DAY EACH WEEK AS YOUR "PROTEIN DAY."

In working with Frankel and Staeheli, I learned that mental activity can change brain structure and function, and *intentional mental activity can change brain structure and function as intended.* In other words, we can change the physical structure of our brains through mental rehearsal just as we can through repeated physical rehearsal. When done properly, mental training is effective because, to a great extent, the effect on the brain is the same whether or not the practice we do is visible to others.

I found out that basketball players who *mentally* practice free throws can improve their performance at least as much as the player who actually spends the same amount of time practicing on the court. *The brain makes no distinction between physical practice and mental practice, so long as the mental training is done effectively.* This realization was important to me. I would need to prepare if I was going to participate in the golf tournament, yet I had little time to physically practice my game.

In the weeks that followed my initial work with Frankel and Staeheli, I discovered how to apply the mental training techniques that had supported countless Portland Health Institute clients to achieve optimal performance under stressful circumstances.

The effort paid off. My medical convention presentation exceeded my expectations. The golf tournament? Not only did I have a wonderful time, I played well enough to help my team win a first place trophy. The strategic planning was equally successful. In fact, the book you're holding is one of the results.

My experiences convinced me beyond any doubt just how powerful the connection between the brain and the body can be.

FOOD for Thought

"If it were easy, everyone would do it."

— William Zinsser

Another Lean for Life Success Story

"The first time I did mental training, I felt a little self-conscious. I had a tough time staying focused. But then I reminded myself that if I had all the answers, I wouldn't be lugging around 75 extra pounds. I had nothing—and everything—to lose by giving it my best shot. I've achieved my goal and am using mental training techniques I learned on the program to train for my first marathon."

THEN & NOW

— *Joshua*

DR. STAMPER

"Is your ketostick
positive? Remember:
You're either in
ketosis or you're
not! If you're not,
make an immediate
adjustment to
correct the situation.
See page 41 for
a quick review."

Anyone can do mental training. At first, you may feel a little self-conscious. Be patient. You'll get better with practice. There's a reason that thousands of people, including athletes, musicians, business professionals, teachers, students, and, yes—dieters—are using this form of mental training. It works!

Now you can learn one more way to strengthen the connection between your brain and body and function more effectively than ever before.

During each Daily Mental Training session, you will be able to:

❏ Intentionally create a peaceful, receptive, undistracted state of mind;

❏ Experience yourself doing those things you've decided are important to you, achieving whatever personal goals you've set and feeling pleased at what you're doing;

❏ Complete the exercise by returning to your usual, alert state of mind, more comfortable and pleased with yourself than before.

DAILY MENTAL TRAINING:
HOW TO DO IT

Choose a quiet place where you can be undisturbed for 15 minutes.

Make yourself comfortable, either lying down or sitting, and close your eyes. If you become aware of any noises or distracting thoughts during your session, simply refocus your attention.

This narration is intended as a guide for creating your own audio tape. Some people read the instructions silently several times, then recreate them in their mind as they do the session. You might also ask a friend or family member to read them to you or to prepare a tape for you.

The following narrative is an abridged version of the MENTORS Daily Mental Training "Inner Mental Room" audiocassette. You may want to use this narrative exactly as written for the first few sessions. With experience, you'll naturally find yourself elaborating in your own way and tailoring it to your needs.

It's helpful to decide what you want to be able to *do*, how you want to be able to *feel,* or how you want to be able to *be* before you begin the session. You can then experience yourself doing it successfully throughout the session. Examples could include: "In this session, I want to...

❑   experience myself at the beach, feeling good about my body."

❑   be calm and focused during my meeting this afternoon."

❑   be able to enjoy the party tomorrow night without letting food be the focus."

You want to experience—in as much sensory detail as you can—doing, feeling, or being whatever you have decided is important to you.

TAPE SCRIPT:

"When you are ready, you will be able to let your attention rest on your breathing. You can experience the air entering your body with each breath in, and you can experience the breath leaving your body every time you breathe out.

If you like, you can let yourself be aware of one part of your body at a time, letting yourself recognize a little bit of tightening, and the sensation of your own strength, as you breathe in... then, as you breathe out, a letting go of whatever tightness you no longer need. You can feel a sensation of comfort and safety.

When you are ready, you can let yourself float down gradually... safe, strong, and comfortable, to a spot from which you can enter your Inner Mental Room. You can let yourself be in your Inner Mental Room, where you know you are safe and secure. You can look around you, and see that you have everything you need. You can arrange your Inner Mental Room exactly as you choose, with whatever furnishings, equipment, and supplies you select.

When you are ready, you can let yourself become aware of a big screen in your Inner Mental Room. On this screen, you can let yourself see the place where you are doing what you are ready to be doing. You can be aware of the time of day, the presence of any people you choose, the details of your surroundings.

You can let yourself hear the sounds of this place ... you can feel the gentle touch of the air on your face, and you can feel what's beneath you, comforting and reassuring. You can let yourself smell the aromas of this place, and even become more aware of the taste in your mouth. When you are ready, you can become aware of yourself, feeling safe, strong, and comfortable. You can let yourself look exactly as you are ready to look, and feel a sense of confidence and satisfaction as you let yourself do what you have decided is important to you...safe and strong and comfortable.

When you are ready, you can let yourself become aware again of being in your Inner Mental Room. You can let yourself return here any time you choose to do the mental training work that you have decided is important to you. Each time you let yourself be in your Inner Mental

"Where the mind dwells, the body tends to follow."

—David Higdon

AFFIRMATIONS

"I am enjoying taking time for myself."

Room, you can feel a deep sense of confidence in your ability to work toward whatever goals you have chosen.

When you are ready, you'll be able to use your breathing in to help you raise your energy level. With each breathing in, you'll be able to become more fully awake and alert, relaxed, and refreshed. And then, when you're ready, you'll be able to breathe in and out two more big breaths, bend and straighten your elbows two times, and again become awake and alert, relaxed, refreshed... able to open your eyes and feel so good all over that you'll be able to feel just...like...smiling!"

THE RIGHT STUFF

Now that you've been exercising regularly for a couple of weeks, you may be thinking about investing in a good pair of walking shoes.

Good walking shoes provide cushioning and support, maximizing comfort and minimizing the risk of injury. Find an athletic shoe store with a knowledgeable sales staff. A good salesperson won't just hand you a box, but will work with you to find the right pair of shoes—one that fits your needs and price range.

ANY QUESTIONS?

Q: *Do Olympic and other world-class athletes really use the kind of mental training techniques I've just learned about?*

A: Absolutely. One of the most high-profile users of mental training techniques is Mike Powell, since 1990 the world's top-ranked long jumper.

Powell's "impossible dream" was to break the world long- jump record set in 1968 in the high, thin air of Mexico City. In early 1991, he began working with Herman M. Frankel, M.D. at Portland Health Institute. Many times each day over the course of seven months, Powell practiced the Daily Mental Training techniques featured in this chapter. He mentally experienced himself jumping successfully in a variety of settings, weather conditions, and stressful situations. He practiced dealing with many different obstacles and distractions. He even mentally rehearsed his physical and emotional state during and after the setting of the new world record.

Powell's efforts paid off in a big way. At the 1991 World Championships in Tokyo, Powell jumped 29 feet, 4$\frac{1}{2}$ inches, shattering track and field's longest-standing record and establishing a new level of human accomplishment.

DAY 17

'WHY ARE YOU DOING THIS TO ME?'

You will learn how to deal successfully with those who try to sabotage your success.

Surprise!" David shouted from the kitchen as Sheila entered the house. "You'll never guess what we're having for dinner."

Sheila didn't need to guess. The aroma of pepperoni pizza was a dead giveaway, and Sheila was not pleased. It was the second time in two weeks that David "surprised" her with a tempting , high-fat, high-carbohydrate indulgence from their favorite Italian restaurant.

"It just doesn't make sense," Sheila said with a shrug. "David tells me he's thrilled that I decided to lose weight. But as soon as I lose a few pounds, he starts undermining my success. I can't help but wonder 'What's going on here?'"

If you've ever tried losing weight before, chances are you understand Sheila's frustration. Perhaps it was your mother who insisted on making her famous homemade pork sausage lasagna. It may have been the workout buddy who told mutual friends how great you're doing but refused to compliment you face to face. Maybe it was your sister, who sent that two-pound box of gourmet chocolates for your birthday even though she knew you were determined to avoid fat and sugar.

You know they love and care about you... so why do they behave in ways that feel more like sabotage than support?

WHAT MOTIVATES DIET SABOTEURS?

By now it should come as no surprise that many people are threatened by change.

In some situations, the people around you may genuinely believe they want you to achieve your goal, yet fear that you—or their relationship with you—may somehow change if you succeed. They prefer the balance and order of your existing relationship—the way things are—over the unknown and the way things might be. This undermines their ability to support you. They become "diet saboteurs," often without realizing what they're doing.

It's also possible that your newfound self-control is making your diet saboteurs feel self-conscious, stirring concerns that if you look better, it will make them look worse. Maybe they're comfortable being the one with the nice body or pretty face while you're the one with the "great personality." Your progress may also be a reminder that they are no closer to their own goals than they were a year ago.

It's important to understand that while diet saboteurs can be maddening, their behavior is seldom premeditated or intentionally cruel. When Sheila asked David, "Why are you doing this to me? Don't you want me to lose weight?" he was dumbfounded. "Of course I do!" he responded.

But Sheila found David's words inconsistent with his recent actions and she told him so. During one of their talks, David eventually acknowledged that perhaps he was feeling "a little threatened" by Sheila's determination to lose the 50 pounds she had gained since their wedding three years earlier.

"He told me it always bothered him when other men used to turn to look at me," Sheila says. "That rarely happened when I was heavier, which suited him just fine. Once we talked about how his inner conflicts were getting in the way of supporting me to achieve something I really wanted, we were able to work it through. Now he's reassured that he's the man for me and I feel better knowing he really has my best interest at heart. We've been walking together every night. What began as a conflict ended up being a real gift to our relationship."

There's an important lesson here. Open, honest communication can cut through the cobwebs of misunderstanding, unspoken feelings, and unresolved conflicts.

DR. STAMPER

"Asking for something greatly increases your odds of getting it."

"The greatest
pleasure in life
is doing what
people say
you cannot do."

—Walter Bagehot

A FOUR-STEP STRATEGY FOR DEALING WITH SABOTEURS

The next time you believe someone is interfering with your weight loss, deal with it directly. Confrontation is rarely necessary, but candor is. This four-step approach will help:

1. *State the problem.* Be specific. Example: "I'm committed to my weight loss program, but it's not always easy. When you offer me potato chips, it only makes it more difficult."

2. *Explain how you feel about the problem and why you need help with the resolution.* Example: "I'm frustrated. I know you care about me, but some of the things you've been doing lately are making it tough. You mean a lot to me and I know this is something we can work through."

3. *Detail what you want.* Don't assume the other person will instinctively know how to provide support. Example: "I'd like it if our time together didn't center on food so often. Instead of meeting for dinner next week, why don't we take in a movie or go for a walk at the park?"

4. *Describe the results you expect and the benefits of your success.* This is an opportunity to reaffirm your goal. Example: "I'm going to feel and look healthier, and I want you to know how much it means to me to know you're supporting me."

Is asking for support always easy? No. But as Sheila will tell you, it's definitely worth the effort.

Your Turn

Who are *your* diet saboteurs? Take a closer look at your relationship with each of the people who came to mind and ask yourself the following questions:

❑ What do you think motivates them to sabotage your weight loss efforts?

❑ Are they usually supportive in other parts of your life?

❑ If so, what can they do—or stop doing—to be more supportive? If they are *never* supportive, what are you getting out of the relationship that motivates you to continue it?

Lean *for* Life®
DAILY ACTION PLAN

Week _____ Day _____ Date _____

Time	Meal Plans	Serving Size	(grams)
_____	**Breakfast**		
	Protein		
	Fruit or Grain		
	Beverage		
_____	**Protein Snack**		
_____	**Lunch**		
	Protein		
	Vegetable		
	Lettuce		
	Fruit		
	Beverage		
	Miscellaneous		
_____	**Protein Snack**		
_____	**Dinner**		
	Protein		
	Vegetable		
	Lettuce		
	Fruit		
	Beverage		
	Miscellaneous		
_____	**Protein Snack**		
		TOTAL	

Keto Reading _____

Weight _____

Vitamins   AM   Noon   PM

Fluids _____

Activities _____
_____
_____
_____

Pedometer Steps _____

WEEKLY BODY MEASUREMENTS

Chest _____ Hips _____

Waist _____ Thighs _____

Abdomen _____

SUCCESS LEARNING TOOLS

Read pages # _____

Audio Tapes _____

Affirmation _____
_____

Plan to Overcome Today's Obstacles:
_____
_____
_____
_____
_____

Notes:
_____
_____
_____
_____
_____
_____

CHOOSE ONE DAY EACH WEEK AS YOUR "PROTEIN DAY."

AFFIRMATIONS

REFOCUSING ON YOUR VISION

Have you looked at your personal Vision Statement since you completed it two days ago? Take time today—and every day throughout your program—to review it until it feels like a part of you. It's also a good idea to revise and update your Vision Statement periodically. Many of the skills you're learning in this book, including affirmations, positive self-talk, and problem-solving strategies, will help support you in achieving your vision.

"I am enjoying my new sense of well-being."

ANY QUESTIONS?

Q: How many mental training sessions should I do each day? I'm very busy.

A: One session a day can make a difference. Even greater benefits will result whenever you can squeeze in a second or third session. Keep track of your mental training work on your Daily Action Plan and observe the results. As long as you're making time for at least one session each day, you'll be in a position to decide how important it is for you to find time to do more.

Q: I'm on the road nearly an hour every day. Why can't I do my MENTORS Mental Training while I'm driving?

A: Unlike other mental training activities you'll be mastering in this program, your MENTORS Mental Training sessions will help you develop an ability to enter a peaceful state of mind, not unlike the state right before you fall asleep. The electrical activity of your brain will differ from that of your normal waking state. In this state, you are free to experience your mental activity and not pay attention to what's going on around you. To drive or operate any machinery could be dangerous to you and others.

YOUR MENTAL BLUEPRINT: WHO—AND HOW—ARE YOU SUPPOSED TO BE?

You can conquer the psychological causes of cravings by redefining your self-image and redrawing your "mental blueprint" of who you are and what you deserve.

For years, Dr. Stamper has believed that losing weight and keeping it off has at least as much to do with what we put in our *minds* as what we put in our *mouths.* That's because how we think and what we expect from—and for—ourselves directly impacts how we eat and how well we take care of our bodies.

As we grew up, we each developed our perspective as to how we—and our lives—were *supposed* to be. Our sense of right and wrong, good and bad, acceptable and unacceptable were influenced by our upbringing, experiences, and social conditioning. This belief system resulted in a "mental blueprint" of who we are and what we think we deserve.

Let's say that your blueprint of your physical self is of a thin, fit person. If so, you're much more likely to stay thin and fit because that's what your blueprint calls for. If you were to start gaining weight, you would be highly motivated to take the necessary steps to lose the

DR. STAMPER

"The most important words you'll ever hear are the ones you tell yourself."

weight, because being fat wouldn't match your blueprint of how you are supposed to be. It wouldn't be "you."

Likewise, if your mental blueprint is of an overweight person, you will be predisposed to do whatever it takes to remain overweight. As long as that blueprint is in place, you will fight to maintain it, *especially if you begin losing weight.* You will be inclined, without realizing it, to sabotage yourself by doing whatever it takes to ensure that your reality resembles your blueprint as closely as possible.

Your blueprint of how things are *supposed* to be influences how things actually *are.* As long as you leave the old blueprint in place, any weight loss or "remodeling" you accomplish isn't likely to last long. Why? Because when you lose weight, your reality will be out of synch with how you are "supposed" to be. Straying too far from your mental blueprint stirs inner conflict.

This reaction has nothing at all to do with being "stupid," "bad," or "stubborn." It has everything to do with being human. When our reality doesn't match our blueprint, we tend to change the reality until it does. By understanding this idea, we can recognize that the problem contains the seeds of the solution.

Let's say, for example, that right this minute you want to eat. You're experiencing cravings and can't identify any physical causes or environmental cues for your sudden urge to eat.

What would happen if you took this opportunity to look at your mental blueprint? Ask yourself the following questions:

- ❏ "What do I think I'm supposed to look like?"

- ❏ "What does my mental blueprint say I'm supposed to be doing in this situation?"

- ❏ "If my mental blueprint shows an overweight person, what might I do in this situation to achieve that blueprint?"

SO WHAT'S THE SOLUTION?

Once you explore these questions, the solution will become obvious—change the blueprint! Replace your "fat" blueprint with a more appropriate one.

You want to fill your mind with images of yourself being energetic, slender, and strong. You want to see yourself moving effortlessly. You want to look at others who have the kind of body you want and see yourself in the same way. You want to identify characters in movies and on television who resemble how you intend to look once you've lost your weight.

Lean *for* Life®
DAILY ACTION PLAN

Week _____   Day _____   Date _____

Time	Meal Plans	Serving Size	(grams)
_____	**Breakfast**		
	Protein		
	Fruit or Grain		
	Beverage		
	_____		
	_____		
	_____		
_____	**Protein Snack**		
	_____		
_____	**Lunch**		
	Protein		
	Vegetable		
	Lettuce		
	Fruit		
	Beverage		
	Miscellaneous		
	_____		
	_____		
_____	**Protein Snack**		
	_____		
_____	**Dinner**		
	Protein		
	Vegetable		
	Lettuce		
	Fruit		
	Beverage		
	Miscellaneous		
	_____		
	_____		
_____	**Protein Snack**		
	_____		
		TOTAL	

Keto Reading _____
Weight _____
Vitamins   AM   Noon   PM
Fluids _____

Activities
_____
_____
_____

Pedometer Steps _____

WEEKLY BODY MEASUREMENTS

Chest _____   Hips _____
Waist _____   Thighs _____
Abdomen _____

SUCCESS LEARNING TOOLS

Read pages # _____
Audio Tapes _____
Affirmation _____
_____

Plan to Overcome Today's Obstacles:
_____
_____
_____
_____
_____
_____

Notes:
_____
_____
_____
_____
_____
_____
_____

CHOOSE ONE DAY EACH WEEK AS YOUR "PROTEIN DAY."

"I am enjoying turning my obstacles into opportunities."

There are more deliberate ways to establish and maintain the blueprint you want. You already have access to a variety of tools that can effectively put new blueprints, patterns, and expectations in place. You know about using BioModifiers to change what's going on inside. You can use powerful positive affirmations to shape your expectations and actions. You can use your mental training sessions to put new images in place.

In the days ahead, you'll learn more ways to change what's inside, so that when you get what you expect, it will be what you really want and you'll be ready to enjoy it.

TELEVISION CAN MAKE YOU FAT

Have you ever grabbed the cookies or potato chips as you tuned in your favorite television show, only to realize later that you almost ate the entire bag?

It's easy to do. When your attention is focused elsewhere, you can be unaware of what—and how much— you're eating. To avoid this trap, limit your eating to one area of your home, preferably your kitchen or dining room table. And when you eat, focus on your meal. Turn off the TV, put down the paper and enjoy the taste, texture, and aroma of the food.

OVERCOMING PLATEAUS

You can overcome temporary stalls and setbacks to achieve your weight loss goal.

Important

The guidelines on pages 43-45 can help you overcome a plateau.

Don't be discouraged if at some point during "Phase 1: Weight Loss," you experience what's commonly known as a weight loss "plateau." A plateau is nothing more than a short period of time, usually one to seven days, during which your body will temporarily resist losing weight. Even though you're in ketosis and following the program carefully, the same number on the scale stubbornly stares back at you.

As you can imagine, plateaus are maddening. After all, most of us believe that if we play by the rules, we'll win. It can be discouraging and demoralizing to do it "right" and not experience the expected payoff.

If you allow them to, plateaus can undermine your self-confidence. They can leave you questioning whether the program "works" and even lead you to overeat out of sheer frustration.

That's why it's so important to understand what plateaus are, why they occur, and how to move beyond them.

"Never give up."

—Winston Churchill

WHAT CAUSES PLATEAUS?

In some cases, plateaus are the result of water retention. If you're retaining water while losing fat, the scale won't necessarily reflect the fat loss. And since water weighs more than fat, it's even possible to lose fat while retaining water and have the scale actually reflect a weight gain.

Some people also experience a plateau whenever they return to a weight to which their body is accustomed. Let's say you started the program weighing 150 pounds and your goal is 125. If you've weighed 135 pounds for years, you may experience a plateau when your body returns to that weight. We refer to this as a "former weight." This kind of "body memory" is common. The body achieves a "comfort zone" that it strives to maintain. No one is certain exactly why this happens, but our experience over millions of treatment sessions tells us it does.

THE GOOD NEWS ABOUT PLATEAUS

All this talk about plateaus may sound pretty grim. But there is good news: *they're only temporary!* It's important to recognize plateaus for exactly what they are. Rather than thinking of them as defeats, derailments, or detours, realize that they're nothing more than temporary road blocks.

Remember:

❑ Plateaus are not permanent.

❑ They are not proof that you "can't lose weight."

❑ Above all, they are no excuse to lose your enthusiasm, momentum, or focus.

IT'S NOT A PLATEAU IF. . .

Now that you understand what a plateau is, it's equally important to recognize what a plateau is not. If you're *not* losing weight and you're *not* in ketosis, you are *not* experiencing a plateau. To convince yourself otherwise is to sabotage your success. *A true plateau occurs only when you are in ketosis and are temporarily not losing weight.*

When you are doing the program correctly, you *will* be in ketosis. Ketosis occurs whenever a person limits his or her carbohydrate intake to between 50 and 100 grams daily. If you're not in ketosis, you're burning carbohydrates—not fat—as your primary energy source.

Those carbohydrates are coming from somewhere. Be honest with yourself. Are you aware of everything you're eating? Read labels carefully to make sure you're not consuming hidden

Lean for Life®
DAILY ACTION PLAN

Week _____ Day _____ Date _____

Time	Meal Plans	Serving Size	(grams)
_____	**Breakfast**		
	Protein		
	Fruit or Grain		
	Beverage		
_____	**Protein Snack**		
_____	**Lunch**		
	Protein		
	Vegetable		
	Lettuce		
	Fruit		
	Beverage		
	Miscellaneous		
_____	**Protein Snack**		
_____	**Dinner**		
	Protein		
	Vegetable		
	Lettuce		
	Fruit		
	Beverage		
	Miscellaneous		
_____	**Protein Snack**		
		TOTAL	

Keto Reading _____
Weight _____
Vitamins   AM   Noon   PM
Fluids _____

Activities _____
_____
_____

Pedometer Steps _____

WEEKLY BODY MEASUREMENTS

Chest _____   Hips _____
Waist _____   Thighs _____
Abdomen _____

SUCCESS LEARNING TOOLS

Read pages # _____
Audio Tapes _____
Affirmation _____
_____

Plan to Overcome Today's Obstacles:
_____
_____
_____
_____
_____
_____
_____

Notes:
_____
_____
_____
_____
_____
_____
_____

CHOOSE ONE DAY EACH WEEK AS YOUR "PROTEIN DAY."

DR. STAMPER

"If you don't take care of your body, where are you going to live?"

carbohydrates. Measure portions. Take special care in maintaining your Daily Action Plan. You may want to do one or two Protein Days until you're back in ketosis, then resume your Weight Loss menu.

If you *are* in ketosis and experiencing a plateau, you may wish to use the Plateau Menu below for *no more than three days* or until you "break" your plateau by losing 1½ pounds or more, whichever comes first.

THE BOTTOM LINE ON PLATEAUS

Stay focused on your goal and remember that plateaus are temporary. Your patience and persistence will pay off. While it's natural to want what you want when you want it, there are times when your body has a mind of its own. Choose to keep your goal in sight.

Important

Continue to have protein snacks while on a plateau.

THE LEAN FOR LIFE PLATEAU MENU

Breakfast

1 egg or egg substitute (boiled, poached, or cooked
    with Pam in a nonstick pan)
½ grapefruit
Choice of any calorie-free beverage

Lunch

3½ ounces, white fish
½ cup, cooked spinach
½ grapefruit
1 cup, lettuce
Choice of any calorie-free beverage

Dinner

3½ ounces, white fish
½ cup, cooked spinach
½ grapefruit
1 cup, lettuce
Choice of any calorie-free beverage

At Bedtime

1 cup, hot lemon water (¼ lemon, boiled in water
    for three minutes)

ANY QUESTIONS?

AFFIRMATIONS

Q: I'm exercising every day and really starting to see and feel results. Exactly what effect does exercise have on my muscles?

A: Exercise changes the way your muscles *work,* the way they *feel,* and the way they *look.* It also improves:

❑   your strength (how much force you can exert; for example, how heavy a load you can carry)

❑   your stamina (how long or how many times you can carry it)

❑   your power (how far you can throw it)

❑   your agility (how gracefully you can move it)

❑   your flexibility (how far you can move it before your joints can't bend or straighten any more)

❑   your coordination (how well you can perform complex moves with it)

❑   your speed (how fast you can move with or without it)

❑   your ability to resist or recover from injury.

When you exercise regularly, your muscles—and you— become firmer and more appealing to look at and touch.

"I am enjoying taking care of myself."

Another Lean for Life Success Story

"On every diet I ever tried, I hit a plateau, got discouraged, and gave up. Lean for Life is the only program that told me up front that plateaus were normal—and that they could be overcome. When I stayed stuck at 201 for four days, I was determined to break through it. And I did! I've been at my lean weight of 185 for nearly two years."

THEN&NOW

— Victor

Your Turn

It's been two weeks since we first looked at how environmental cues can trigger a desire to eat even when we're not hungry.

When was the last time you found yourself eating in response to an external cue such as a TV food commercial, a particular pastry shop, or the company of certain people?

_____

_____

What did you eat? _____

_____

How did you feel afterward? _____

_____

What could you have done instead? _____

_____

What did you learn? _____

_____

AFFIRMING THE POSITIVE

You can communicate with yourself in ways that affirm your ability to achieve your goals.

Have you ever had one of those truly perfect days when you felt capable, confident, and totally self-assured? You were ready for any challenge that came your way and felt thoroughly equipped to accomplish whatever you set your mind to. Those nagging inner voices—the ones that sometimes insist "I can't do this" or "I'm not good enough"—were nowhere to be heard.

You can have more of those days by using a simple but effective technique called affirmations. In just a few minutes every day, you can neutralize the effects of negative thinking on your mind and body, replacing them with a soothing, encouraging, optimistic way of thinking and feeling that will make your life more positive and successful.

Affirmations are positive, personal statements that you create, write down, and repeat to yourself to affirm, in your mind, that you're capable of accomplishing your goal.

ACCENTUATE THE POSITIVE

Effective affirmations highlight your *positive behavior* by stating what you are doing rather than not doing. Example: "I am eating

DR. STAMPER

"Negative thoughts are like pebbles. If you carry one or two around, you may not notice. But when you accumulate enough of them, they really weigh you down."

healthy foods that nourish my body" rather than "I am not eating junk food anymore." They also highlight your *positive feelings* by describing what you want rather than what you don't want. Example: "I am becoming healthy, strong, and lean" rather than "I don't want to be fat anymore." What's more, they also underscore your *positive commitment* by focusing on firm statements ("I am succeeding at becoming Lean for Life") rather than tentative or predictive statements ("I hope to become Lean for Life").

An easy way to remind yourself of the positive foundation of affirmations is to visualize yourself moving actively and happily toward what you want instead of running away from what you don't want.

At first, the notion of being able to enhance your self-confidence by making positive statements about yourself may sound like little more than New-Age psychobabble. But while "the power of positive thinking" may be a cliche, the fact is positive thinking *can* be powerful! Research suggests that affirmations can have a significant psychological impact on our emotions and health by neutralizing the unconscious negative beliefs and feelings that undermine so many people's success.

WHEN TO DO AFFIRMATIONS

Many of our patients recite an affirmation before they get out of bed in the morning and in the evening as they prepare to fall asleep. That way, the affirmation is the first and last message they hear each day. These are the times when you're most likely to be in a relaxed, receptive state of mind. In order for the affirmation to become a routine part of your thinking, it's necessary to experience it in a deeper, more "whole body" kind of way rather than merely on a "thinking" level.

An affirmation that comes from your heart will always be appropriate for you, even when you're asserting something that doesn't feel quite real yet. If you deliver the message to yourself often enough, it will begin to feel real. And that's the point. You make a choice as to how you want to be and then help yourself become that person.

Lean *for* Life®
DAILY ACTION PLAN

Week _____   Day _____   Date _____

Time	Meal Plans	Serving Size	(grams)
_____	**Breakfast**		
	Protein		
	Fruit or Grain		
	Beverage		
_____	**Protein Snack**		
_____	**Lunch**		
	Protein		
	Vegetable		
	Lettuce		
	Fruit		
	Beverage		
	Miscellaneous		
_____	**Protein Snack**		
_____	**Dinner**		
	Protein		
	Vegetable		
	Lettuce		
	Fruit		
	Beverage		
	Miscellaneous		
_____	**Protein Snack**		
	TOTAL		

Keto Reading _____
Weight _____
Vitamins   AM   Noon   PM
Fluids _____

Activities _____
_____
_____

Pedometer Steps _____

WEEKLY BODY MEASUREMENTS

Chest _____   Hips _____
Waist _____   Thighs _____
Abdomen _____

SUCCESS LEARNING TOOLS

Read pages # _____
Audio Tapes _____
Affirmation _____
_____

Plan to Overcome Today's Obstacles:
_____
_____
_____
_____
_____
_____

Notes:
_____
_____
_____
_____
_____
_____

CHOOSE ONE DAY EACH WEEK AS YOUR "PROTEIN DAY."

Food for Thought

Your Turn

"You never lose until you stop trying."

—Mike Ditka

As you prepare to create your affirmations, remember that they are always personal "I" statements. That's because they're about you and no one else. Also be sure that your affirmations are stated in the present tense. Say "I am..." rather than "I will..." and you will come from a position of having already achieved your stated desire.

Now that you have an understanding of affirmations and how you can benefit from using them, it's your turn to come up with some you can use. These sample affirmations may spark some ideas:

- ❏ "I have everything I need to be healthy."
- ❏ "The food I'm eating makes me healthy and lean."
- ❏ "I feel wonderful when I exercise."
- ❏ "I am filled with energy."
- ❏ "I am a problem solver."
- ❏ "I can handle whatever challenges life gives me."
- ❏ "I am proud of myself for being a patient, kind person."
- ❏ "I am enjoying becoming Lean for Life."
- ❏ "I am having fun being active."
- ❏ "I am becoming healthy, strong, and lean."
- ❏ "I am smiling."
- ❏ "I am sticking with my program."

Write three affirmations on a sheet of paper. Revise them until they feel right to you. Do they highlight your positive feelings? Do they encourage positive behavior? Do they affirm your positive commitment? Are they "I am" statements?

Once you're satisfied with your affirmations, write them here:

Affirmations

1. _____

2. _____

3. _____

Starting today, choose one of your affirmations and repeat it throughout the day. The more often you repeat your affirmation, the more it will become a part of you and the way you see the world.

VISUALIZATIONS: WHAT YOU GET IS WHAT YOU SEE

You can learn to diffuse negative self-talk
by visualizing your success.

Ask anyone who knows William and they'll tell you he's one of the nicest people you'd ever want to meet. And he is—to everyone but himself.

While he's understanding and easy-going with his wife, children, friends, and employees, the 42-year-old landscaper never realized how hard he was on himself. Then one morning, his Lindora nurse suggested he write down every negative thought he had and every negative comment he made about himself for the rest of the day.

By noon, William's list already included: 9:26AM: "I really blew it!" ... 10:15AM: "At the rate I'm going I'm never going to lose these last 10 pounds!" ... 10:38AM: "Gee, I'm about as sharp as a marble!" ... 11:20AM: "What a klutz!" ... 11:55AM: "I'm absolutely terrible at remembering names!"

The exercise was quite an eye-opener. William suddenly realized how unforgiving and judgmental he was with himself—totally different from the way he was with loved ones, friends, or even casual acquaintances.

William's not unique. Many of us surrender undeserved power to our negative inner voices. What's more, while we're quick to label our "failures" as being "bad" or "stupid," we're rarely as willing to give ourselves credit when things go well.

In fact, some of us react to our successes as harshly as we do our setbacks, dismissing our accomplishments ("I was lucky"), minimizing our achievements ("It was no big deal"), and even predicting future failure ("I never do things right twice in a row—I'll probably mess up tomorrow!"). When was the last time you said to yourself, "I did that exactly the way I wanted to and it was terrific?"

While this kind of negative self-talk may not sound damaging, it takes a toll. What we say to ourselves tends to be a predictor of what will actually happen. The steady drip of negative messages can eventually wash away our self-esteem and confidence in our ability to function effectively in the world.

Recognizing how you talk to yourself is important because *what you say to yourself in any particular setting has a profound effect on how you are likely to perform in that setting in the future.* When you tell yourself something often enough, you begin to believe it. You begin to "see" it in your mind.

The scenes you play in your head change your brain structure. These scenes are examples of BioModifiers, those things we do on purpose to help ourselves get what we want by changing what's happening inside our brains. As the scene that you visualize and store in your brain becomes more and more familiar, it will begin to play itself out that way more predictably and more often, because you will start functioning in the ways that have become more familiar to you.

That's why many world-class athletes and classical musicians include mental rehearsal of their routines and emotions prior to a competition or performance. They also mentally replay the details of their successes after every event, mentally revising imperfect moments so that what gets stored in their memories is a successful execution of the task rather than an unsuccessful one.

You can learn how to use the same kind of powerful, brief visualizations for specific purposes. Whether you're preparing to exercise, about to enter a restaurant, or contemplating a decision, you can pause briefly to visualize the scene exactly as you would like to see it play out, complete with sound, sensation, aroma, taste, and emotion.

A brief visualization differs from a Daily Mental Training session or other mental training in that it's shorter and can take place when you're fully alert. It's totally focused on one scene and is typically done immediately before you begin or resume an activity in your everyday life. A brief visualization may be used as a positive response to negative

Lean *for* Life®
DAILY ACTION PLAN

Week _____   Day _____   Date _____

Time	Meal Plans	Serving Size	(grams)
_____	**Breakfast**		
	Protein		
	Fruit or Grain		
	Beverage		
_____	**Protein Snack**		
_____	**Lunch**		
	Protein		
	Vegetable		
	Lettuce		
	Fruit		
	Beverage		
	Miscellaneous		
_____	**Protein Snack**		
_____	**Dinner**		
	Protein		
	Vegetable		
	Lettuce		
	Fruit		
	Beverage		
	Miscellaneous		
_____	**Protein Snack**		
	TOTAL		

Keto Reading _____
Weight _____
Vitamins   AM   Noon   PM
Fluids _____

Activities _____
_____
_____

Pedometer Steps _____

WEEKLY BODY MEASUREMENTS

Chest _____   Hips _____
Waist _____   Thighs _____
Abdomen _____

SUCCESS LEARNING TOOLS

Read pages # _____
Audio Tapes _____
Affirmation _____
_____

Plan to Overcome Today's Obstacles: _____
_____
_____
_____
_____
_____
_____

Notes: _____
_____
_____
_____
_____
_____
_____
_____

CHOOSE ONE DAY EACH WEEK AS YOUR "PROTEIN DAY."

self-talk because it replaces a negative pattern with an emotionally positive one. Similarly, brief visualizations can be used immediately after you've experienced a disappointment or failure, or immediately before starting a challenging activity.

Brief visualizations can be done at any time. They don't require time alone, closing your eyes, or entering an alterative state of consciousness. They simply require that you remind yourself of your power to create the positive mental state that leads to success.

Go ahead. Do it. See what happens.

"I feel terrific when I eat nutritious, healthy food."

THE HIDDEN PAYOFFS OF BEING FAT

If you had asked Colleen a year ago to tell you about the benefits of being fat, she would have denied there were any.

But today—after losing 109 pounds and gaining a greater sense of awareness—the 32-year-old entertainment attorney knows better.

"Not only did I drop the weight, but I dropped the defenses that helped make me fat in the first place," she explains. "There were benefits I wasn't even aware of until I had to give them up. My weight was a convenient excuse for anything that wasn't working in my life. If I lost a case, for example, I would tell myself it was because the jury didn't like fat women. One day it dawned on me—my fat was taking a toll on my self-respect as well as on my body."

Several months into her program, Colleen also came face-to-face with a truth she had long denied: for 10 years she had been using her fat to insulate herself from men.

"I was never comfortable with all of the attention I got from boys in high school," she explains. "The more weight I put on, the less of a problem it was. Without my realizing it, this was my way of protecting myself. At that point in my life, it never occurred to me that I could be a thin, attractive woman and not be hassled or harrassed by men."

What have been *your* hidden payoffs for being overweight? One of the main themes of this book is awareness. By clearly identifying benefits you derived from being overweight, you will take an important first step toward ensuring that you don't lapse into self-defeating patterns of behavior.

THE POWER OF PRACTICE

You will learn how consistency, repetition, and practice can help you maintain the results you've achieved.

It's a joke as old as New York's Empire State Building: A tourist approaches a Manhattan street musician near Central Park and says, "Excuse me, sir, how do I get to Carnegie Hall?"

As the musician's bow dances across the strings of his violin, he grins and replies, "Practice, my friend, practice!"

As tired as it is, this joke illustrates a relevant point: to maintain any degree of success, you must *keep* doing what you've been doing to achieve the results you're currently enjoying.

It all boils down to "use it or lose it," a cliche that also happens to be an absolute truth. As renowned pianist Artur Rubenstein once observed, "If I miss one day, I can tell; if I miss two days, the audience can tell."

Like Rubenstein, you need to keep up with your daily regimen, too. By doing moderate exercise, you'll maintain the increased mitochondria and increased insulin receptors you've built up in your muscle cells.

It's equally important that you continue your mental training. It results in specific changes in the circuits of connections among brain cells and in brain chemistry that will work to your advantage.

"No one lives
forever. But if
you do it well,
once is enough."

—Dr. David Viscott

And just like physical training, in which many athletes cross-train by blending strength training, flexibility training, and speed training into an overall regimen, mental training is also "cross-trainable."

Since you have a variety of mental training tools available to choose from—including positive affirmations Daily Mental Training sessions, your personal Vision Statement, Motivator cards, and brief visualization techniques—you have plenty of opportunities to do different kinds of mental training without the process ever becoming boring or tedious.

So keep it up! You've invested too much to get where you are to run the risk of returning to where you were!

ACTIVITY BY THE NUMBERS

Ever wonder how many calories you were burning while standing, swimming, or shoveling snow?
With this chart, you'll know.

Calories Burned During 15 Minutes of Activity

Activity	125 lbs.	175 lbs.	250 lbs.
Sleeping	15	21	30
Standing	18	24	36
Walking (4 mph)	78	108	153
Climbing stairs	219	303	432
Cycling (13 mph)	133	186	267
Washing windows	52	72	103
Shoveling snow	97	133	195
Light office work	37	51	75
Carpentry	48	66	96
Chopping wood	90	126	181
Basketball	87	123	175
Dancing (vigorous)	72	99	141
Golfing	49	72	102
Racquetball	112	156	216
Water skiing	90	132	195
Swimming (crawl)	60	84	120
Volleyball	64	97	141

Lean *for* Life®
DAILY ACTION PLAN

Week _____ Day _____ Date _____

Time	Meal Plans	Serving Size	(grams)
_____	**Breakfast** _____		
	Protein		
	Fruit or Grain		
	Beverage		
_____	**Protein Snack**		
_____	**Lunch**		
	Protein		
	Vegetable		
	Lettuce		
	Fruit		
	Beverage		
	Miscellaneous		
_____	**Protein Snack**		
_____	**Dinner**		
	Protein		
	Vegetable		
	Lettuce		
	Fruit		
	Beverage		
	Miscellaneous		
_____	**Protein Snack**		
		TOTAL	

Keto Reading _____
Weight _____
Vitamins   AM   Noon   PM
Fluids _____

Activities _____
_____
_____

Pedometer Steps _____

WEEKLY BODY MEASUREMENTS

Chest _____   Hips _____
Waist _____   Thighs _____
Abdomen _____

SUCCESS LEARNING TOOLS

Read pages # _____
Audio Tapes _____
Affirmation _____
_____

Plan to Overcome Today's Obstacles:
_____
_____
_____
_____
_____
_____

Notes:
_____
_____
_____

CHOOSE ONE DAY EACH WEEK AS YOUR "PROTEIN DAY."

"I enjoy my exercise."

EXERCISING YOUR OPTIONS: MAKING FITNESS FUN

After you've done anything for a few weeks, your initial enthusiasm can begin to fade. But your exercise routine doesn't have to be routine at all. Here are three tips to help you stay moving and motivated:

1. **Set short-term goals.** Whatever your ultimate fitness goal happens to be, you're more likely to achieve it if you divide it into smaller, less imposing intermediate goals. Rather than committing to an hour of exercise, five times a week for the next year, focus instead on the present and the immediate future. What are you realistically willing and able to commit to during the next two weeks? Thirty minutes? Forty? Three times a week or four? Write your commitment down and then do it. Keep a written record of your exercise accomplishments in a notebook. During this two-week period, assess your exercise and activities and renew your commitment to the process.

2. **Schedule exercise into your day.** Whenever you make a business, social, or medical appointment, you probably write it down in your calendar. You consider it a commitment and you don't want to forget. As you begin your fourth week of the program, think of your exercise time as an appointment with yourself. Schedule it in just as you would a dental appointment or dinner with a friend—and then keep the date!

3. **Remember that when it comes to exercise, anything is better than nothing.** No matter how stressed, busy, or exhausted you are, it's important that you exercise—even if only for a brief time. Make a deal with yourself that on your scheduled workout days, you'll squeeze in at least a light, 20-minute workout, no matter what.

   Be resourceful. This might mean taking a brisk walk through the airport as you wait for a flight. It could mean stretching in your office while returning phone calls or using your coffee break as an exercise break. Instead of strolling down to the cafeteria, go outdoors for a brisk 10-minute walk. Take the stairs instead of the elevator. Rather than circling for a close parking space, park your car in the first space you see and walk to your destination.

Any movement is better then none, so do what you can. The more demanding your day, the more valuable this break will be.

A HEALTHY INVESTMENT

You will learn to identify the "ingredients" you consider important for a healthy life.

If you were asked to share your "recipe" for a healthy life, which essential "ingredients" would top your list?

As you begin your last week of Weight Loss, it's a question well worth asking—and answering. Before you read any further, take a few minutes and write down what you consider to be the basic components of a healthy, balanced life:

_____

_____

_____

_____

_____

_____

Our years of clinical experience have taught us that certain "ingredients" are essential. How does your list compare to this one, which was developed with our friends at Portland Health Institute?

H   Higher purpose

E   Eating healthy food

A   Activity that is moderate and regular

L   Laughter and play

T   Time alone

H   Human contact

Higher purpose. People who feel more fulfilled are those who live with a sense of purpose and passion, commit to ideas and ideals greater than themselves, and give of themselves without expectation of personal gain. What do *you* believe in? What stirs your passions? How often do you lend your time and talent to causes and concerns that matter to you?

Eating healthy food. Even though you're currently in the Weight Loss phase of the program, your ultimate goal is to develop a healthy way of eating that will serve you well for the rest of your life. As you know, the emphasis is on plenty of fruits and vegetables, protein for energy and muscle building, moderate carbohydrates, and little fat. Once you've lost all the weight you want to lose, you'll see the benefits of moderation and common sense in maintaining your weight loss.

Activity that is moderate and regular. Activity is vital in the life of anyone who truly wants to live well. We're only beginning to understand how our miraculous bodies manage to function so beautifully. But one thing we do know is that the human body was designed for movement, and all of our mental and physical systems

THE BUDDY SYSTEM

You might be surprised to discover how willing one of your friends, neighbors, or co-workers would be to join you in your exercise routine. The support and structure that the "buddy system" offers will keep both of you motivated. It's easy to break promises to yourself. But when you know someone is waiting for you at the gym or at the beginning of your walking trail, you're much more likely to show up. And when you do, you both benefit!

Lean *for* Life®
DAILY ACTION PLAN

Week _____ Day _____ Date _____

Time	Meal Plans	Serving Size	(grams)
_____	**Breakfast**		
	Protein		
	Fruit or Grain		
	Beverage		
_____	**Protein Snack**		
_____	**Lunch**		
	Protein		
	Vegetable		
	Lettuce		
	Fruit		
	Beverage		
	Miscellaneous		
_____	**Protein Snack**		
_____	**Dinner**		
	Protein		
	Vegetable		
	Lettuce		
	Fruit		
	Beverage		
	Miscellaneous		
_____	**Protein Snack**		
		TOTAL	

Keto Reading _____

Weight _____

Vitamins   AM   Noon   PM

Fluids _____

Activities _____
_____
_____

Pedometer Steps _____

WEEKLY BODY MEASUREMENTS

Chest _____ Hips _____

Waist _____ Thighs _____

Abdomen _____

SUCCESS LEARNING TOOLS

Read pages # _____

Audio Tapes _____

Affirmation _____

_____

Plan to Overcome Today's Obstacles:

_____
_____
_____
_____
_____

Notes:

_____
_____
_____
_____
_____
_____

CHOOSE ONE DAY EACH WEEK AS YOUR "PROTEIN DAY."

"Every worthwhile accomplishment, big or little, has its stages of drudgery and triumph; first the beginning, then a struggle, then a victory."

—Anonymous

depend on keeping our bodies in good working order. Is your body getting enough movement?

Laughter and play. When we laugh, our bodies work better, our relationships work better, and our work works better. Henry Wheeler Shaw once commented that "laughter is the sensation of feeling good all over and showing it principally in one place." Not only does a good laugh feel good, it *does* good. Laughter is one of the ultimate BioModifiers. It helps nurture the soul. A sense of humor and an ability to play can be true lifesavers even in the darkest times. We need to remind ourselves to balance the serious with the playful. When was the last time you told a joke? Flew a kite? Walked in the rain? Surprised a friend or loved one with a relaxing day trip?

Time alone. "If one sets aside time for a business appointment or shopping expedition," Anne Morrow Lindbergh once observed, "that time is accepted as inviolable. But if one says, 'I cannot come because that is my hour to be alone,' one is considered rude, egotistical, or strange. What commentary on our civilization."

As the pace of contemporary life seems to ever-accelerate, it's easy to forget what Lindbergh clearly realized—that time alone is time well spent. Solitude allows the soul time to reflect upon itself. There is an emotional clarity and inner calm that can occur only when we're alone, reflecting and thinking without interruption. Thomas Edison suggested that "the best thinking has been done in solitude; the worst has been done in turmoil." When we hop off life's treadmill for some "alone time" every now and then, we recharge the spirit and renew our sense of wonder and joy in life. When is the last time you spent a quiet afternoon alone, with no radio, reading, or rules? Do you do it as often as you'd like? Why not?

Human contact. The connection to others through words and touch is life itself. We are made for it. And when we don't get enough of it, we tend to become depressed and sick more often. Fortunately, we all possess the power to initiate and maintain contact with the world around us. How good are you at staying connected?

Are your "HEALTH" needs currently being met in ways you find satisfying? In which of these six categories do you feel most fulfilled? Which could use a little more attention?

Take time to treat yourself well. "HEALTH" is an investment in yourself. And like any good investment, it will pay off.

ANY QUESTIONS?

AFFIRMATIONS

Q: *I'm doing moderate exercise every day but I don't like it. Any suggestions?*

A: There's a big difference between activity not being your favorite thing and being something you truly dread. Try defining what it is about exercise that you don't like.

Be specific. Is it having to shower afterward? Maybe you could walk first in the morning before you shower and get ready for work. Is it lonely? What not invite a friend to come along? Is it the weather? You could always drive to a nearby shopping mall and walk there. Is it boring? Take along a portable audio tape or CD player with headphones and listen to lively music or a motivational tape. Vary your routine or try something new. What specific solutions can you think of for overcoming your discomfort?

It's possible that no solutions will come to mind or will feel right. Under these circumstances, you can remind yourself that exercise is valuable, even on those days when you don't feel like doing it. This gives you the freedom to address the question, "Is it OK for me to do something I don't like if I have reason to think it will help me achieve my goals?"

Review your Motivator cards whenever you feel yourself losing momentum and motivation. This will help you shift your focus to why you're doing the program and how much you enjoy the benefits.

"I appreciate my body and feel good about the changes I see."

DAY 24

SUCCESS STRATEGIES: MEETING 'REAL LIFE' CHALLENGES

You will discover simple but effective strategies for successfully managing the temptations that life presents.

No matter how motivated and determined you are to stick with your plan to lose weight, there are going to be times when "real life" presents situations that heighten temptation and lower your resistance.

But that doesn't suggest you have to become a victim of circumstance. By anticipating everyday challenges and approaching them with a Plan of Action, you can sidestep the predictable pitfalls that derail many dieters.

Today and tomorrow, we'll take a look at a number of potentially difficult "real life" situations—everything from grocery shopping to ordering in restaurants to eating on the run—and offer practical strategies to help you stay focused on results. First, let's discuss one of the biggest traps—and how to avoid falling into it.

MARKETING 101

A trip to your neighborhood grocery store can be a true test of will. They're strategically designed to stimulate impulse buying, and their marketing tactics work. There are, however, ways you can level the playing field the next time you go shopping:

Review your Motivator card. Before you go food shopping, review your reasons for becoming Lean for Life. This will help you stay focused and motivated.

Never shop when you're hungry. Always eat a meal or a protein snack first.

Avoid shopping when you're stressed and/or tired. The more frazzled you are, the more likely you'll be to buy impulsively. If you're used to shopping on your way home from work, try going either early in the morning when you're rested or later at night after you've had dinner and time to relax.

Steer clear of your "danger zones." For some, that may be the store bakery. For others, it's the aisle stocked with nuts, potato chips, and other salty snacks. You know your danger zones better than anyone. By avoiding them, you'll reduce the temptation to buy "a little bag" of this or "just one box" of that.

"If you have the will to win, you have achieved half your success. If you don't, you have achieved half your failure."

—David Ambrose

"MR. MITO" SAYS:

"Ever heard of the Toothbrush Tush Push or the Towel Toner? They're "bonus" exercises you can do in your bathroom while getting ready in the morning. Like most exercises, they're more fun when you do them to music.

❑ *Toothbrush Tush Push: The music's playing and there's toothpaste on the brush. Stand tall with your feet apart and your toes turned out. As you brush, bend and then straighten your knees to the music. Who would have ever guessed that good oral hygiene could also result in a firmer rear end?*

❑ *Towel Toner: Stand with your feet apart. Grab a towel with both hands, then raise your arms above your head and pull the towel taught. Bend from side to side, at least 12 times each. Make it fun by getting with the beat of the music.*

Sure, they sound silly—but extra exercises like these can eventually result in bonus benefits you can see!"

Serving sizes are stated in both household and metric measures, and reflect the amounts people actually eat.

Calories from fat are shown on the label to help consumers meet dietary guidelines that recommend people get no more than 30 percent of their calories from fat.

The list of nutrients covers those most important to the health of today's consumers, most of whom need to worry about getting too much of certain items (fat, for example), rather than too few minerals, as in the past.

%Daily Value shows how a food fits into the overall daily diet.

The label now tells the number of calories per gram of fat, carbohydrates, and protein.

Some daily values are maximums, as with fat (65 grams or less); others are minimums, as with carbohydrates (300 grams or above). The daily values on the label are based on a daily diet of 2,000 and 2,500 calories. Individuals should adjust the values to fit their own calorie intake.

Nutrition Facts

Serving Size ½ cup (114g)
Serving Per Container: 4

Amount Per Serving

Calories 90   Calories from Fat 30

	% Daily Value*
Total Fat 3g	5%
Saturated Fat 0g	0%
Cholesterol 0 mg	0%
Sodium 300mg	13%
Total Carbohydrate 13g	4%
Dietary Fiber 3g	12%
Sugars 3g	
Protein 3g	

Vitamin A 80% • Vitamin C 60% • Calcium 4% • Iron 4%

*Percent Daily Values are based on a 2,000 calorie diet. Your Daily Values may be higher or lower depending on your calorie needs:

Nutrient		2,000 Calories	2,500 Calories
Total Fat	Less than	65g	80g
Sat Fat	Less than	20g	25g
Cholesterol	Less than	300mg	300mg
Sodium	Less than	2,400mg	2,400mg
Total Carbohydrate		300g	375g
Fiber		25g	30g

Calories per gram:
Fat 9   •   Carbohydrates 4   •   Protein 4

Learn to read food labels. Labeling reforms mandated by the Food and Drug Administration have made food labels much more "user friendly" but they can still be confusing. Take a look at the food label above. What would you say is the percentage of fat?

If you answered five percent, you'd be making a very common error. Take a closer look at the "Calories from Fat." Each serving contains 90 calories, and 30 of those calories are from fat. That means this food is *33% fat!* The "Total Fat" percentage of five percent simply indicates that a single serving of this food provides five percent of the daily value, *based on a 2,000 calorie diet.*

Always shop from a list. If it's not on your list, don't buy it. This simple strategy will save you time, money, and unwanted calories.

Lean *for* Life®
DAILY ACTION PLAN

Week _____ **Day** _____ **Date** _____

Time	Meal Plans	Serving Size	(grams)
_____	**Breakfast**		
	Protein		
	Fruit or Grain		
	Beverage		
_____	**Protein Snack**		
_____	**Lunch**		
	Protein		
	Vegetable		
	Lettuce		
	Fruit		
	Beverage		
	Miscellaneous		
_____	**Protein Snack**		
_____	**Dinner**		
	Protein		
	Vegetable		
	Lettuce		
	Fruit		
	Beverage		
	Miscellaneous		
_____	**Protein Snack**		
		TOTAL	

Keto Reading _____

Weight _____

Vitamins   AM   Noon   PM

Fluids _____

Activities _____

_____

_____

Pedometer Steps _____

WEEKLY BODY MEASUREMENTS

Chest _____ Hips _____

Waist _____ Thighs _____

Abdomen _____

SUCCESS LEARNING TOOLS

Read pages # _____

Audio Tapes _____

Affirmation _____

_____

Plan to Overcome Today's Obstacles: _____

_____

_____

_____

_____

_____

Notes: _____

_____

_____

_____

_____

_____

CHOOSE ONE DAY EACH WEEK AS YOUR "PROTEIN DAY."

AFFIRMATIONS

"I am in control of
what I eat."

Shop less and buy more. The more often you visit the market, the more likely you are to buy food you don't need.

Buy fresh. When buying fruits and vegetables, remember that fresh is better than frozen, and frozen is better than canned.

Beware of misleading buzzwords. Food manufacturers are well aware that the American consumer is more health conscious today than ever before. It's no coincidence that so many food products are now being marketed as "Lite", "Low-Fat," and "Reduced Calorie." These products often deliver exactly what they promise and represent tasty alternatives to their higher-fat counterparts. But in some cases, the so-called "healthy" alternatives are as loaded with fat and sugar as the original products they pretend to improve upon.

Know what you're buying. Compare labels. "Lite" as opposed to what? "Lower in calories" than what? "Reduced" from what? Avoid becoming a victim of shrewd food marketing by shopping smart!

Tomorrow, we'll look at a number of other "real life" situations—and how you can successfully face the challenges they present.

PUT YOUR MONEY WHERE YOUR MOUTH IS

A Michigan State University study found that people who bet $40 they could stick with their workout program for six months had a whopping 97% success rate. Only 20% of those who didn't make the bet followed through on their program. Challenge your workout buddy. The first one to slack off pays up!

TAKING THE OFFENSIVE: OVERCOMING OTHER 'REAL LIFE' TEMPTATIONS

You'll learn how to neutralize five everyday danger zones and stay focused on your goal.

While that trip to the grocery store can be a tormenting test of self-control and willpower, it's certainly not the only "real life" situation that can jeopardize your success.

Today let's focus on five other situations in which temptation looms large. By using a combination of the 20 success strategies offered here, you can neutralize temptation's impact and stay focused on your weight loss goal.

HAVE IT YOUR WAY

Whoever said eating in restaurants has to be an ordeal just because you're on a weight loss program? In fact, you can learn how to turn dining out into an enjoyable, stress-free event. Here are some of the success strategies our patients find most helpful:

Choose restaurants carefully. If you're not sure whether a restaurant serves chicken or fish, call ahead and ask. Avoid "all you can eat" buffets and restaurants known for huge portions. It'll be much easier for you to stick with your program if you're not sitting

"People can be divided into three groups: those who make things happen, those who watch things happen, and those who wonder what happened."

—Yiddish Proverb

across from a friend who's devouring the "Mother Lode" mega-platter of nachos.

Speak up. If a friend or business associate suggests meeting at a restaurant where you think you might have a tough time ordering food you can eat, don't hesitate to suggest alternatives: "I'd love to meet you for lunch, but instead of pizza, let's try that new seafood restaurant down the street." You'll discover that most people are fairly flexible, especially if you tell them why you're making your suggestions.

Avoid temptation by avoiding the menu. That's right—don't even read it. Instead, tell the server exactly what you would like. Surprisingly, this is just as easy to do in inexpensive coffee shops and chain restaurants as it is in elegant five-star establishments. The restaurant business is extremely competitive, and most restaurants are more than willing to satisfy health-conscious customers by preparing food to order.

Be specific when ordering. If you want your entree broiled, baked, or grilled, be sure to say so. Ordering what you want might sound something like this: "I'd like a skinless chicken breast, grilled or broiled, some steamed vegetables without butter, and a small green salad with vinegar on the side." If it's not prepared properly, have them try again.

Steer clear of the dessert tray. If you're sure that a restaurant typically presents a dessert tray, tell your server before you finish your entree that you won't be having dessert. If you'd like fresh fruit, ask what is available. Again, it's a matter of planning ahead and exercising control.

Always keep an "emergency supply" of protein snacks in your briefcase, car, and office. If you find yourself in a dining situation where it's truly impossible to order well, order light and satisfy your hunger later with a protein snack.

NOW YOU'RE COOKING

You can create delicious meals for yourself and your family while you're becoming Lean for Life. In fact, you'll probably find that food tastes better, because you'll be preparing it in healthier ways. Make a point to:

Prepare only one evening meal. Period. If you cook one meal for your family and another for yourself, you'll likely end up feeling

Lean *for* Life®
DAILY ACTION PLAN

Week _____ **Day** _____ **Date** _____

Time	Meal Plans	Serving Size	(grams)
_____	**Breakfast**		
	Protein		
	Fruit or Grain		
	Beverage		
_____	**Protein Snack**		
_____	**Lunch**		
	Protein		
	Vegetable		
	Lettuce		
	Fruit		
	Beverage		
	Miscellaneous		
_____	**Protein Snack**		
_____	**Dinner**		
	Protein		
	Vegetable		
	Lettuce		
	Fruit		
	Beverage		
	Miscellaneous		
_____	**Protein Snack**		
	TOTAL		

Keto Reading _____
Weight _____
Vitamins   AM   Noon   PM
Fluids _____

Activities
_____
_____
_____

Pedometer Steps _____

WEEKLY BODY MEASUREMENTS

Chest _____ Hips _____
Waist _____ Thighs _____
Abdomen _____

SUCCESS LEARNING TOOLS

Read pages # _____
Audio Tapes _____
Affirmation _____
_____

Plan to Overcome Today's Obstacles:
_____
_____
_____
_____
_____
_____

Notes:
_____
_____
_____
_____
_____
_____

CHOOSE ONE DAY EACH WEEK AS YOUR "PROTEIN DAY."

DR. STAMPER

"You are responsible. You are in control. You possess the power to stay focused on your goal and achieve it."

deprived. Instead, make healthy, tasty meals that are on your program and can also be enjoyed by the entire family. Not only will you reduce your time in the kitchen, you'll also be including your family in a healthier way of eating.

Obesity tends to run in families—not only because of genetics, but because bad eating habits are often learned early in life. By encouraging your children to eat in more healthy ways, you can help them avoid many of the food-related challenges you find yourself facing today.

Delegate food-related duties. If you have children, have them help at mealtime. Younger children can set and clear the table. Older kids can help you prepare a salad.

Don't turn meals into a power struggle. Even the most health-conscious kids are not always going to want to eat what you're eating on the program. If they're old enough, let them prepare their own dinners once a week. Perhaps you can plan dinner out once a week so that everyone in the family can order what he or she wants.

Stick with the choices and portion sizes designated on your program. Just because some family members eat larger portions or have additional foods doesn't mean you have to. Don't let anyone else's appetite affect your success!

THE MORNING RUSH

A healthy breakfast is a great way to start the day, yet it's the meal that dieters are most likely to skip. No matter how busy you are, you can enjoy breakfast and still get to work on time:

Make time for it. Build breakfast into your morning—even if it means getting up 10 minutes earlier.

Plan ahead. Boil a dozen eggs at one time so you have plenty to last through the week. A few minutes before you walk out the door, drop a slice of bread in the toaster or take a piece of fruit and a container of nonfat yogurt out of the refrigerator, and pour yourself a cup of coffee. As you're heading to work, you can enjoy an easy-to-make breakfast that's much less expensive and better for you than the fast-food alternatives.

UNDER THE WEATHER?

Flu, colds, viruses, and other illnesses can take a real toll on your body. This is especially true whenever you're eating less food than normal. Since your body perceives any illness as a threat, it conserves energy (calories) and water in an effort to help you recuperate.

This basic biological fact can temporarily stall your weight loss efforts. Don't get discouraged or distracted. Make getting well and feeling better a priority and continue on your program unless otherwise directed by your physician. As you begin feeling better, you'll overcome any temporary weight plateaus that you've experienced while recuperating.

Whenever you're not feeling well, be sure to:

Call or visit your doctor. Discuss your symptoms.

Carefully read labels on all over-the-counter medications. Choose pressed cold tablets such as Dristan or Comtrex. Many liquid medications and throat lozenges contain sugar and/or alcohol, both of which tend to stimulate appetite. They're loaded with extra calories, too.

Continue taking vitamins. Your daily supply of vitamins contains 600 mg. of Vitamin C, 10 times the U.S. recommended daily allowance.

Drink plenty of water and herbal teas. Make a point to stay hydrated even if you're not thirsty.

Don't skip meals. No matter how dull your appetite may be, it's essential that you get enough to eat—especially when you're not feeling well.

EATING ON THE JOB

It's happened to all of us. You're at work and you don't have time to get away for lunch. Those vending machines in the break room or cafeteria may seem like a quick fix—and they are. The problem, of course, is that a *quick* fix isn't always a *healthy solution*. But with a little advance planning, eating at work can be every bit as easy—and delicious—as eating at home:

Take your lunch. What better way to plan ahead—and guarantee that what you want will be available—than to make your own? If your workplace doesn't have a refrigerator you can use, carry your food in a small cooler. If you have access to a microwave, take prepared lunch entrees in plastic containers.

Don't skip your three daily protein snacks. Make a habit of taking your mid-morning and mid-afternoon snacks with you every morning. Keep a diet soda and a couple of protein snacks handy.

"Love yourself first and everything else will fall into line. You really have to love yourself to get anything done in this world."

—Lucille Ball

"I am in charge of what I eat, when I eat, and how much I eat."

Make healthy choices when ordering fast food. If a quick trip to a nearby fast-food restaurant is your only option, be cautious and think ahead. When you're hungry, it's easy to order impulsively and then regret it an hour later. Most fast-food places serve salads, and many offer char-broiled or grilled chicken. You can always order the grilled chicken sandwich and skip the bun.

No matter *where* you eat, the choice to eat well is always yours.

ANY QUESTIONS?

Q: *Does it matter what time of day I walk?*

A: What matters more than *when* you walk is *that* you walk. There is no one "right" time. The benefits you enjoy can vary depending on the time of day. Consider the "four S's" when deciding what's best for you:

❑ *Schedule.* When does your walk best fit into your schedule? When are you most likely to do it and enjoy it? When you plan an evening walk, do you usually do it or do you sometimes talk yourself out of it? If so, you'd probably be better off walking in the morning.

❑ *Safety.* Do you feel safe walking your favorite routes at the times that are best for you? Is there another place or a different time in which you'd be safer?

❑ *Sun exposure.* Schedule your walks with sun exposure and temperature in mind. Some people love the solar power that comes with the heat of the day. Others burn easily and find that too much sun saps their energy. Do whatever works for you—just be sure to protect your skin with sunscreen.

❑ *Side benefits.* Do you prefer the energizing benefits of an early-morning walk or the relaxing opportunity to unwind that results from walking at the end of the day? Many people find that a late-morning walk helps curb their appetites, while others value the "second wind" they get from walking mid-afternoon. Decide which "side benefits" are most important—and treat yourself to at least one dose a day.

GO WITH THE 'FLOW'

*You will learn about one of the rewards
of engaging in activities such as exercise
with commitment and concentration.*

Imagine an experience so joyous and exhilarating that you would
pursue it regardless of the obstacles, costs, or risks. While engaged in
this adventure, feelings of self-doubt or self-consciousness would be
nonexistent. You would be oblivious to time, and your concentration
would be so total that you wouldn't worry or think about anything else.

Sound like a ticket you'd buy? An adventure you'd empty your
savings account for? A dream you'd pursue? What if I told you that you
could achieve this experience through physical activity? That's right.
Physical activity. If you've been exercising regularly, you may have
already experienced this remarkable state of mind that athletes and
other achievers refer to as "flow."

Flow was first identified by University of Chicago psychologist
Mihaly Csikszentmihalyi. In his book *Flow: The Psychology of Optimal
Experience* (Harper & Row, 1990), Csikszentmihalyi describes this
internal state as "so enjoyable that people will do it even at great cost,
for the sheer joy of doing it," one in which people "are so involved in an
activity that nothing else seems to matter."

Lean *for* Life®
DAILY ACTION PLAN

Week _____   Day _____   Date _____

Time	Meal Plans	Serving Size	(grams)
_____	**Breakfast**		
	Protein		
	Fruit or Grain		
	Beverage		
_____	**Protein Snack**		
_____	**Lunch**		
	Protein		
	Vegetable		
	Lettuce		
	Fruit		
	Beverage		
	Miscellaneous		
_____	**Protein Snack**		
_____	**Dinner**		
	Protein		
	Vegetable		
	Lettuce		
	Fruit		
	Beverage		
	Miscellaneous		
_____	**Protein Snack**		
		TOTAL	

Keto Reading _____

Weight _____

Vitamins   AM   Noon   PM

Fluids _____

Activities _____

_____

_____

Pedometer Steps _____

WEEKLY BODY MEASUREMENTS

Chest _____   Hips _____

Waist _____   Thighs _____

Abdomen _____

SUCCESS LEARNING TOOLS

Read pages # _____

Audio Tapes _____

Affirmation _____

_____

_____

Plan to Overcome Today's Obstacles:

_____

_____

_____

_____

_____

_____

Notes:

_____

_____

_____

_____

_____

_____

CHOOSE ONE DAY EACH WEEK AS YOUR "PROTEIN DAY."

This state of mind has been studied in artists, factory workers, musicians, athletes, surgeons, homemakers, Buddhist monks, even a Japanese Hell's Angels motorcycle gang. Regardless of age, gender, ethnicity, cultural background, or type of activity, Csikszentmihalyi and his colleagues found the same pattern in people who are fully engaged in what they are doing—"a state of complete involvement and satisfaction."

Flow experiences rarely result from passive activities such as watching television. They are much more likely to occur when people do something that stretches their capacities, something that requires the full concentration of their abilities.

In a flow state, there's a perfect balance between the level of the challenge and your level of skill. The immediate consequence is that you are fully engaged in the activity. You're unburdened by any awareness of time, external distractions, the quality of your performance, and even yourself.

Flow is the experience that prompts people to think, "This is as good as it gets!" Your problems vanish and fresh solutions surface. You experience a liberating sense of harmony and safety that frees you to function more fully than before.

If you haven't felt it yet, stay active and interested. Before long, you're bound to experience the rush that results when you "go with the flow."

AFFIRMATIONS

"I appreciate my body and feel good about the changes I see."

IT SURE WORKED FOR THEM!

Albert Einstein, Charles Dickens, and Frank Lloyd Wright each knew the value of exercising their bodies as well as their minds. They were all inveterate walkers, often seen strolling through their neighborhoods during breaks from their respective work in physics, literature, and architecture.

While no one knows how often Webster went walking, you've got to love his definition of exercise: "the act of bringing into play or realizing in action; to use." After all, that's exactly what exercise is—*using* your body and realizing results through action!

Regular walks certainly seemed to work for these creative geniuses. Are you giving them a chance to work for you?

DAY 27

Today's Eating Plan

If you're participating in a clinical program, your health care professional may determine it's appropriate for you to extend your Weight Loss module by up to 4 more weeks. Otherwise, you'll begin Metabolic Adjustment tomorrow.

PREPARING FOR 'METABOLIC ADJUSTMENT'

You will learn more about the next part of the program: how it works and how you'll benefit from doing it successfully.

Over the past month you've faced—and met—many challenges. You've had the opportunity to use new skills in overcoming obstacles. You've learned to be successful at losing weight. You're looking and feeling healthier than you did just four weeks ago. You're now ready to be successful at the greatest challenge of all—preparing to *maintain* the weight loss you've achieved.

Whether you're close to your goal or still have a way to go, you'll begin "Metabolic Adjustment" in just a couple of days. During this vital 14-day portion of the program, you will begin eating more food, making additions according to a specific schedule. You'll also continue maintaining your Daily Action Plan, exercising daily, and using the mental training techniques you find most helpful.

During Metabolic Adjustment, *the goal isn't to lose weight, but to gradually eat more and increase your metabolism without gaining weight.*

THE BENEFITS OF 'METABOLIC ADJUSTMENT'

During Metabolic Adjustment, your body will:

DR. STAMPER

❑ adjust to the fact that it has recently lost a significant amount of body fat, so that it will not start working desperately to replace it as soon as you begin to eat more calories.

❑ adjust your body chemistry back to a state in which you're not in ketosis and you are able to eat more carbohydrates again.

❑ raise your metabolic rate so that you're burning more calories and are able to eat more food without gaining weight.

"What your mind can conceive, your body can achieve."

❑ physiologically begin the process of adjusting your setpoint to your new, lower weight so you can enjoy eating enough so you're not hungry but not so much that you'll regain weight.

❑ restore the normal physiological pattern of using carbohydrate as well as fat for fuel.

Metabolic Adjustment is a time to take stock and take pride in what you've accomplished. It's also a time to stay focused.

Even though it's straightforward and easy to follow, "Metabolic Adjustment" is the part of the program in which people are most likely to make mistakes and interrupt their success.

Once you've completed this two-week process, you'll have a decision to make. You can either begin a second Weight Loss series (of up to four weeks) or, if you've achieved your goal weight, you'll advance to the second phase of the program: Lifetime Maintenance.

MINI GOALS = MAJOR CHANGES

What will you accomplish *today*? For the next week, focus on one element of the program and challenge yourself to achieve a specific "mini-goal" every day, such as:

❑ logging 3,000 more steps on your pedometer.
❑ drinking 10 glasses of water.
❑ repeating an affirmation six times a day.

You'll soon find that you've effected a major change in how you feel and look. Remind yourself of your "mini-goal" several times during the day, and be sure to follow through. The sense of accomplishment you'll feel when you achieve it will keep you motivated.

Lean *for* Life®
DAILY ACTION PLAN

Week _____ Day _____ Date _____

Time	Meal Plans	Serving Size	(grams)
_____	**Breakfast**		
	Protein		
	Fruit or Grain		
	Beverage		
_____	**Protein Snack**		
_____	**Lunch**		
	Protein		
	Vegetable		
	Lettuce		
	Fruit		
	Beverage		
	Miscellaneous		
_____	**Protein Snack**		
_____	**Dinner**		
	Protein		
	Vegetable		
	Lettuce		
	Fruit		
	Beverage		
	Miscellaneous		
_____	**Protein Snack**		
		TOTAL	

Keto Reading _____

Weight _____

Vitamins   AM   Noon   PM

Fluids _____

Activities _____
_____
_____

\# Pedometer Steps _____

WEEKLY BODY MEASUREMENTS

Chest _____ Hips _____

Waist _____ Thighs _____

Abdomen _____

SUCCESS LEARNING TOOLS

Read pages # _____

Audio Tapes _____

Affirmation _____
_____
_____

Plan to Overcome Today's Obstacles:
_____
_____
_____
_____
_____
_____

Notes:
_____
_____
_____
_____
_____
_____

CHOOSE ONE DAY EACH WEEK AS YOUR "PROTEIN DAY."

ANY QUESTIONS?

Q: *I find that walking really perks me up when I'm feeling depressed. It also calms me down when I'm feeling anxious. How does my body know which way to react to the same activity?*

A: Getting "perked up" and "calmed down" may sound like movement in opposite directions, but think of them as moving toward the center, where mind and body are in balance. Walking and other moderate exercise can also:

❏ raise or lower your energy level, depending on whether you were feeling sluggish or overexcited when you started.

❏ help you become more alert or help you get ready for sleep, depending on whether you're just waking up or ending a long, full day.

Q: *Why is it that I often find it easier to open up and have a meaningful discussion with someone when we're walking than when we're sitting across a table from one another?*

A: Many people find that when they're physically active and moving in a continuous, easy rhythm, it's easier for them to think more clearly and communicate more openly. In this state, resistance is lowered and feelings of self-consciouness seem to diminish. If you're someone who derives these added benefits from walking, enjoy and make good use of it!

"I have confidence that I will succeed."

DAY 28

THE PAST IS A PRESENT AS YOU PROCEED TO THE FUTURE

You'll focus on discoveries you've made and declare your intentions for applying them as you move into the next part of Phase 1.

Today's Eating Plan

If your health care professional has determined it's appropriate to extend your Weight Loss module, you'll continue following the Weight Loss guidelines and re-read Days 1-26. Otherwise, begin Metabolic Adjustment today.

Congratulations! Today you will complete the Weight Loss module of your Lean for Life program. You now stand at the gateway of "Metabolic Adjustment," ready to begin a 14-day period in which you'll learn how to gradually begin eating more food without regaining the weight you've just lost.

During the past four weeks, you've learned how to take care of yourself in new ways. You've acquired valuable new tools and discovered new approaches, strategies, and ideas for losing weight and improving your health. Every day of the Weight Loss module has been designed to empower you, to help you increase your awareness and knowledge, and to support you in taking greater responsibility for your body and your life.

Over the past four weeks you've undertaken a challenging personal journey. In the process, you've charted new territory; some days were undoubtedly more stimulating or stressful than others. But like the pieces of a puzzle, they ultimately fit together to create a finished product.

As you pause before beginning the next part of your trip, it's time to take stock, to decide which tools and strategies you've found most useful in developing and maintaining your focus and commitment over the past four weeks. In other words, what newfound knowledge and awareness will be most valuable as you advance to "Metabolic Adjustment" and then on to "Phase 2: Lifetime Maintenance"?

We know from clinical experience that the people who continue to integrate the concepts of the program into their lives are the ones most likely to succeed at maintaining their weight loss. That's why today is devoted to looking back—and to focusing on how you can continue benefitting from your recent discoveries as you as move ahead.

SOLIDIFYING YOUR SUCCESS

The following exercise is one most people find fun and easy to do.

There are no right or wrong answers. What matters most is that you answer the questions thoughtfully. You may want to read each question, think about it for a few minutes, review the book briefly to refresh your memory, and consider all the ideas that come to mind. Then open your eyes and write down your answer.

1. **The most important thing I want to remember about *my eating* and weight loss is:**

   _____

   _____

   I can apply this in my life in the following ways:

   _____

   _____

2. **The most important thing I want to remember about *my exercise* and weight loss is:**

   _____

   _____

   I can apply this in my life in the following ways:

   _____

   _____

Food for Thought

"There is no upper limit to what individuals are capable of doing with their minds... There is no obstacle that cannot be overcome if they persist and believe."

— E. F. Wells

"The important thing is not where you were or where you are, but where you want to get."

—Dave Mahoney

3. **The most important thing I want to remember about** *my mental attitude* **and weight loss is:**

_____

_____

I can apply this in my life in the following ways:

_____

_____

4. **The most important thing I want to remember about** *my emotional health* **and weight loss is:**

_____

_____

I can apply this in my life in the following ways:

_____

_____

5. **The most important thing I can do to** *take care of myself* **as I continue my program is:**

_____

_____

I can apply this in my life in the following ways:

_____

_____

As you prepare to advance to Metabolic Adjustment, let yourself reflect on the rewards you're enjoying as a result of your efforts. What changes do you most notice in your body? How do you look and feel today, compared to four weeks ago? Have the changes you're making in your body affected how you feel about yourself and how you relate to others?

Whatever benefits you're enjoying are enhanced by the fact you've earned them yourself. The progress you've made is a direct result of *your* actions, your willingness to set a goal and make it happen. In the process, you've demonstrated remarkable commitment and determination. You've invested energy, enthusiasm, and effort in the program and in yourself—and it's paying off. This will continue as long as *you* continue.

The first phase of this program has helped many thousands of people achieve their goal of becoming Lean for Life. The second phase of the program has helped them succeed in *staying* Lean for Life.

Let them do the same for you!

"MR. MITO" SAYS:

"How many steps have you logged on your pedometer today? Did you know a report from the Office of the Surgeon General cautions that a "lack of physical activity is detrimental to your health"?

It's true. And guess what it recommends? A minimum of 30 minutes a day of moderate exercise. So step to it!"

MEASURING UP

It's that time again! Measure your chest, waist, lower abdomen, hips, and upper thigh, and jot down the numbers below. How do they compare to the measurements you took back on Prep Day 2?

Chest _____   Hips _____

Waist _____   Thigh (upper) _____

Lower Abdomen _____

Lean *for* Life®
DAILY ACTION PLAN

Week _____   Day _____   Date _____

Time	Meal Plans	Serving Size	(grams)
_____	**Breakfast**		
	Protein		
	Fruit or Grain		
	Beverage		
_____	**Protein Snack**		
_____	**Lunch**		
	Protein		
	Vegetable		
	Lettuce		
	Fruit		
	Beverage		
	Miscellaneous		
_____	**Protein Snack**		
_____	**Dinner**		
	Protein		
	Vegetable		
	Lettuce		
	Fruit		
	Beverage		
	Miscellaneous		
_____	**Protein Snack**		
		TOTAL	

Keto Reading _____
Weight _____
Vitamins   AM   Noon   PM
Fluids _____

Activities
_____
_____
_____

Pedometer Steps _____

WEEKLY BODY MEASUREMENTS

Chest _____   Hips _____
Waist _____   Thighs _____
Abdomen _____

SUCCESS LEARNING TOOLS

Read pages # _____
Audio Tapes _____
Affirmation _____
_____

Plan to Overcome Today's Obstacles:
_____
_____
_____
_____
_____
_____
_____

Notes:
_____
_____
_____
_____
_____

CHOOSE ONE DAY EACH WEEK AS YOUR "PROTEIN DAY."

Thanks to the ever-powerful mind-body connection, the most influential words you'll ever hear are the ones you speak to yourself.

Back on Day 12, you completed an exercise in which you became more familiar with the voices that form your "Inner Committee." Which have been most vocal lately? Take a few minutes to think about the messages your various inner voices convey—and how they affect you.

When was the last time you heard from your Frightened Voice?

_____

What was the message?

_____

What impact did it have on you?

_____

When was the last time you heard from your *Angry Voice?*

_____

What was the message?

_____

What impact did it have on you?

_____

When was the last time you heard from your *Critical Voice?*

_____

What was the message?

_____

What impact did it have on you?

_____

continued

"I am enjoying the results of my efforts and energy!"

AFFIRMATIONS

"The world is
for those who
make their dreams
come true."

— Harold Gray

When was the last time you heard from your *Joyful Voice?*
_____

What was the message?
_____

What impact did it have on you?
_____

When was the last time you heard from your *Curious Voice?*
_____

What was the message?
_____

What impact did it have on you?
_____

When was the last time you heard from your *Loving Voice?*
_____

What was the message?
_____

What impact did it have on you?
_____

When was the last time you heard from your *Confident Voice?*
_____

What was the message?
_____

What impact did it have on you?
_____

Remember: Speak nicely to yourself. Your brain hears you!

METABOLIC ADJUSTMENT

*You will be able to eat more food
without gaining weight.*

Anyone who has ever dieted knows that *losing* weight is only the first step. The challenge is keeping it off—and that's exactly what Metabolic Adjustment and Lifetime Maintenance are designed to help you accomplish.

After *every* four-week Weight Loss module you choose to do, you will move on to Metabolic Adjustment. During this 14-day period, your goal will be to increase your body's metabolism, the rate at which you burn calories, by gradually increasing the amount of food you eat—without experiencing any weight gain.

Why, you may be wondering, is adjusting your metabolism so important? Whenever your body is forced to work on a reduced number of calories, as it's been doing during the Weight Loss module, it eventually adapts and trains itself to live on whatever calories it's getting—*without* losing weight. This built-in survival mechanism is called "metabolic adaptation." It's your body's way of protecting you against starvation. While metabolic adaptation can be a real lifesaver if you're stranded without food in the middle of nowhere, it can be a source of enormous frustration when you're eager to continue losing weight.

"Metabolic Adjustment" is a vital part of the program. It's also one of the most easily misunderstood. Many people—especially those who haven't yet achieved their Lean for Life goal—resist doing this phase of the program. And it's easy to understand why. After all, if you're still losing weight and you want to lose more, you want to keep doing what's working for you. It's easy to rationalize that taking a break from weight loss and adding new foods will only delay your progress.

In fact, the opposite is true. If you fail to complete this important part of the program, you may soon find it difficult, if not impossible, to lose more weight. You may manage to lose a few "bonus pounds," but you'll lose them much more slowly. And before you know it, you're likely to regain those pounds—and more—whenever you begin eating more food.

If you *have* achieved your weight loss goal, you may find yourself resisting Metabolic Adjustment for different reasons. If you've lost all the weight you wanted to lose, it's easy to think that you've crossed the finish line, that you've succeeded. And you have—at least partially. But what you haven't done yet is taken the steps necessary to *maintain* your weight loss.

When you fail to adjust your metabolism, you set yourself up for a frustrating fall. That's because once you begin adding foods that are not part of Phase 1—or begin eating greater quantities of food—you will tend to gain weight rapidly because your body hasn't had a chance to adjust to the intake of extra "fuel." What it can't burn it stores as fat for future use. Even if you substitute foods that contain the same number of calories, you run the risk of decreasing your muscle mass and increasing your fat percentage. As a result, you may look and feel larger, even though your weight hasn't changed.

It's important for you to understand that the purpose of Metabolic Adjustment is *not* to lose weight, but to readjust your body's ability to metabolize an increasing number of calories. Since weight loss is not the goal of Metabolic Adjustment, you will not be in ketosis during this part of your program. You will, however, continue doing one "Protein Day" each week for weight control, focus, and discipline.

Metabolic Adjustment is an easy-to-follow process. The instructions for each of the three levels are very specific. Each level builds upon the one before it. Your menu choices are identical to those on Weight Loss.

As the chart on the next page illustrates, the difference between the Metabolic Adjustment and Weight Loss menu is that *some of your portion*

METABOLIC ADJUSTMENT

LEVEL 1 **(Days 1-3)**	**LEVEL 2** **(Days 4-7)**	**LEVEL 3** **(Days 8-14)**
BREAKFAST		
2 Proteins	2 Proteins	2 Proteins
1½ Fruit or Grain	1½ Fruit or Grain	1½ Fruit or Grain
1 Beverage	1 Beverage	1 Beverage
PROTEIN SNACK		
LUNCH		
1½ Proteins	2 Proteins	2 Proteins
1 Vegetable	1 Vegetable	1 Vegetable
Lettuce (unlimited)	Lettuce (unlimited)	Lettuce (unlimited)
1 Fruit	1 Fruit	1 Fruit
2 Misc.	2 Misc.	1 Grain
1 Beverage	1 Beverage	2 Misc.
		1 Beverage
PROTEIN SNACK		
DINNER		
1½ Proteins	2 Proteins	2 Proteins
1 Vegetable	1 Vegetable	1 Vegetable
Lettuce (unlimited)	Lettuce (unlimited)	Lettuce (unlimited)
1 Fruit	1 Fruit	1 Fruit
2 Misc.	2 Misc.	1 Grain
1 Beverage	1 Beverage	2 Misc.
		1 Beverage
PROTEIN SNACK		

sizes are increased. The only addition of a new food during Metabolic Adjustment occurs on Day 8, when you'll begin adding a Grain serving at both lunch and dinner.

Your menu will continue to emphasize lean protein choices. Protein with each meal is essential to avoid triggering a carbohydrate/insulin

Another Lean for Life Success Story

"All my life people have called me stubborn. But I've always denied it because I am, of course, incredibly stubborn. I never realized exactly how bullheaded I could be until I lost, regained, lost, regained, and lost the same 20 pounds in less than two years! How did I do it? Skip Metabolic Adjustment and you'll find out for yourself.

"Every time I achieved my weight loss goal, I figured I was home free. Even after I regained and lost the weight a second time, I convinced myself I could do it my way, that Metabolic Adjustment and the Lifetime Maintenance phase were only for other people. I, of course, was 'special.'

"One day I was feeling very frustrated and made some comment to the effect that the program didn't work. Eva, my Lindora nurse, wasn't buying it. She pointed out that the Weight Loss module of the program had worked for me not once but three times, and that Metabolic Adjustment and Phase 2 hadn't 'worked' because I hadn't done them.

"As stubborn as I sometimes am, even I had to admit that Eva had a point. My problem wasn't with the program. It was my resistance to following directions, following through, and committing 100%. I realized I'd cheated myself out of a lot of benefits of the program, among them lasting results.

"Eva encouraged me to think of Metabolic Adjustment as a step toward achieving 'metabolic fitness.' I continued exercising regularly and followed the three levels. Once I fully committed to doing it, I found I was able to tolerate more calories without gaining weight. I was also more satisfied with my meals and less tempted to snack.

"It's been nearly two years since I finished Metabolic Adjustment. During that time, I've maintained my 20-pound weight loss. Do I feel better physically? You bet. But what feels just as terrific is finally breaking free from a pattern that was leading to nothing but frustration."

—Fran

response, which can make you hungry and increase your likelihood of bingeing.

You will begin with Level 1, increasing quantities at breakfast, lunch, and dinner as indicated on page 219. When you've increased food quantities as indicated on Level 1 and have maintained your weight within 1½ pounds (based on your weight when you began Metabolic Adjustment,) you'll move on to Level 2, repeating the same process before continuing to Level 3. Once you have gradually made these food changes over 14 days—and maintained your weight within 1½ pounds—you will have completed "Metabolic Adjustment."

Any time you experience a weight gain of 1½ pounds or more, have a Protein meal—substitute a Protein choice from the menu for your dinner *that evening*. The extra weight should be gone the next day. You may need to do this for more than one day if you seriously overate. Do not move on to the next level of food addition until your weight is back within the 1½ pound range.

What makes 1½ pounds the "magic number"? First, your body weight can fluctuate that much for any number of reasons, so becoming concerned over a weight gain of a half-pound or even a pound can be much ado about nothing. The 1½-pound marker also establishes a clear guideline that will help you keep a minor fluctuation from becoming a major weight gain. No one gains 20, 30, or 50 pounds overnight. It sneaks up on you, a pound or two at a time. That's why weighing yourself daily is as important during Metabolic Adjustment as it was during Weight Loss. When you step on the scale every morning, you'll know exactly where you stand.

If, during Metabolic Adjustment, you find it difficult to stay within the 1½-pound guideline, you're probably either eating too much of your menu foods, eating food that's not included on the menu, and/or not exercising enough to burn the number of calories you're consuming. Review your Daily Action Plan to make sure you're following the levels correctly and consuming enough protein. And, as always, monitor your level of activity.

Your success will come faster and easier if you resist the urge to alter the program in any way. Tens of thousands of people have learned to become Lean for Life *by following the program through both phases*. It works! Eat all three meals and your protein snacks—including all of the food additions specified on your program—even if you're "not hungry." (If you don't eat them, you soon will be.)

You've already succeeded in losing weight during the first module of your program. Once your metabolism is elevated, you'll be ready to either begin another Weight Loss cycle or move into the final phase: Lifetime Maintenance.

DR. STAMPER

"Remember to weigh yourself daily and correct for any 1½-pound gain. Do not move on to the next level of food additions until you have completed each level without a weight gain."

Your Turn

Staying motivated during the Weight Loss portion of the program is easy because every day you see and feel the benefits. You "see the reward." *Staying motivated to maintain your weight, however, is more of a challenge.* You don't get to see or feel the progress.

That's why it's important for you to decide what your personal rewards for maintaining your weight loss "look like." In other words, what are the payoffs you are enjoying as a result of your maintaining your weight loss? By clearly identifying the specific benefits, you'll be more likely to sustain your motivation.

The following list includes a sampling of the benefits Lindora patients have described for maintaining their weight loss:

❏ "I can wear my favorite clothes without holding my stomach in."
❏ "I can run, bend, and jump without excess fat getting in the way."
❏ "For the first time in 10 years, both my blood pressure and cholesterol levels are normal."
❏ "I can tie my shoes without getting short of breath."
❏ "I no longer feel self-conscious about my body when I go to the beach."
❏ "My arthritis doesn't flare up as often because I'm not putting as much stress on my joints."
❏ "I recently had a physical and my doctor told me I'm in better shape now than I was four years ago."
❏ "I look and feel healthier than I did in college."

What "rewards" are you enjoying now that you've lost weight? Ask friends and family if they've noticed any other perks. You'll probably be surprised by what they say. List all the benefits and payoffs that come to mind:

_____

_____

_____

Update and review this list every day during Metabolic Adjustment. Focusing on the benefits of maintaining your weight loss will motivate and remind you that maintaining is as important as losing.

SUCCESS STRATEGIES: 12 WAYS TO GUARANTEE RESULTS DURING METABOLIC ADJUSTMENT

During Metabolic Adjustment, it's important that you:

1. *Eat three meals a day.* We've already discussed why it's so vital to make all your food additions as outlined on your program. It's equally important that you eat three meals a day, every day. Because you've become used to eating less during your Weight Loss module, you may find yourself tempted to occasionally skip meals. Don't do it! You need to continue to reinforce the healthy patterns that you established during Weight Loss.

2. *Maintain your Daily Action Plan.* Your Daily Action Plan will help you stay aware of what, when, where, why, and how much you're eating. Be sure to keep an accurate written record of everything you eat and drink. That way, if you experience any weight gain, you can review your record to determine what happened and know how to correct it.

3. *Weigh yourself each morning.* Continue this important habit.

4. *Listen to your Lean for Life audio tapes.* Every time you do, you'll discover new insights about the program—and yourself.

5. *Practice your affirmations.* The goal, of course, is to stay motivated and focused on reinforcing your healthy self-image.

6. *Exercise and monitor the number of steps you take.* There are countless physical and psychological payoffs to moderate exercise: It increases your mitochondria, elevates your mood, boosts your metabolism, burns calories, tones and firms your body, and helps you feel more relaxed and less hungry. Continue to walk or do some other form of moderate exercise at least five days a week.

7. *Take your vitamin and mineral supplements.* They help maximize absorption and utilization of the food you eat, and guard against nutritional deficiencies.

8. *Do one Protein Day every week.* We recommend a weekly Protein Day because it helps control your appetite and provides a structure of self-discipline that will benefit you as you move toward Lifetime Maintenance. It's best to designate one day each week—preferably Monday—as your Protein Day. That way, you start your week off with a clear focus on your program and your progress.

DR. STAMPER

"If you find yourself
regaining weight,
skip your evening
meal and have only
the protein portion.
Take charge.
Take control."

9. ***Drink at least 80 ounces of water or other calorie-free fluid every day.*** Liquids—especially water—keep you hydrated, control appetite, and eliminate excess fluids.

10. ***Avoid sugar, alcohol, hydrogenated fat, animal fats, and white flour.*** Why? Here's a quick recap:

Sugar is not only loaded with empty calories, but it takes your system on a roller-coaster ride that ends with a dip in blood sugar and results in cravings.

When you eat sugar or high-carbohydrate foods, your body must produce insulin in the pancreas for you to utilize the concentrated carbohydrate calories. The insulin flows into your bloodstream to move the carbohydrates—which are now in the form of glucose—into the cells for use as energy. When this process occurs, your blood sugar drops. The result? You get hungry and crave carbohydrates. Protein, on the other hand, is metabolized more slowly, allowing your blood sugar to remain more stable and your appetite to remain in check. The bottom line: The less sugar you eat, the better off you'll be.

Alcohol not only contains empty calories, but it also inhibits fat metabolism and self-control. If you choose to drink, stick with white wine or a wine spritzer and limit your consumption. Caution: You may find that because you've avoided alcohol during the Weight Loss module of your program, you have a diminished tolerance and one drink now has the same effect as two or three. Be careful.

White flour and the baked goods that contain it are typically higher in carbohydrates and fat. They tend to promote weight gain and trigger cravings. Whole grains are healthier, and they taste better, too.

Hydrogenated fat and animal fats—butter, regular margarine, solid cooking fat, and coffee creamers are artery cloggers loaded with unwanted calories. Choose unsaturated, nonhydrogenated fats, such as olive oil.

Having completed the Weight Loss module of your program, you've already reduced or eliminated these foods from your diet. You've taken some major steps forward. Why take even one step back?

11. ***Have a protein snack as needed to control cravings.*** Whenever you're overcome by a "snack attack," have a protein-enhanced snack and a large glass of water. Keep protein snacks handy—in your glove compartment, at work, in your purse, or pocket. That way, you always have a healthy choice available.

12. ***Stay focused.*** Metabolic Adjustment only takes two weeks. Stick with it—the results are worth it!

"MR. MITO" SAYS:

"The more you listen, the more you lose! Preliminary evidence from studies at the University of Wisconsin suggest that listening to motivational tapes can—and does—affect one's weight. In one study, participants raised their metabolic rates simply by listening to guided imagery tapes that helped them focus on revving up their metabolism."

ANY QUESTIONS?

Q: *Why should I care about Metabolic Adjustment? What's in it for me?*

A: No one ever goes on a weight loss program believing "I'm going to lose 30 pounds and then gain it back!" They think "Once I lose the weight, I'll be fine—I'm never going to be fat again!"

But the truth is most people who diet—some experts suggest as many as 95%— regain all their weight within five years. That's why the focus of Lean for Life isn't simply on losing weight. It's maintaining your weight loss that ultimately makes the difference. *Metabolic Adjustment is a valuable and necessary part of this process.*

Lean *for* Life®
DAILY ACTION PLAN

LEVEL 1 METABOLIC ADJUSTMENT

Week ___I___ Day ___I___ Date _____

Time	Meal Plans	Serving Size	(grams)
____	**Breakfast**		
	Protein	2	
	Fruit or Grain	1½	
	Beverage	1	
____	**Protein Snack**		
____	**Lunch**		
	Protein	1½	
	Vegetable	1	
	Lettuce	Unl.	
	Fruit	1	
	Beverage	1	
	Miscellaneous	2	
____	**Protein Snack**		
____	**Dinner**		
	Protein	1½	
	Vegetable	1	
	Lettuce	Unl.	
	Fruit	1	
	Beverage	1	
	Miscellaneous	2	
____	**Protein Snack**		
		TOTAL	

Weight _____

Vitamins   AM   Noon   PM

Fluids _____

Activities _____
_____
_____

Pedometer Steps _____

WEEKLY BODY MEASUREMENTS

Chest _____ Hips _____
Waist _____ Thighs _____
Abdomen _____

SUCCESS LEARNING TOOLS

Read pages # _____
Audio Tapes _____
Affirmation _____
_____

Plan to Overcome Today's Obstacles:
_____
_____
_____
_____
_____
_____

Notes:
_____
_____
_____

CHOOSE ONE DAY EACH WEEK DURING METABOLIC ADJUSTMENT
AS YOUR "PROTEIN DAY." DO YOUR "PROTEIN DAY" EXACTLY
AS YOU DID DURING WEIGHT LOSS.

Lean for Life®
DAILY ACTION PLAN

LEVEL I METABOLIC ADJUSTMENT

Week __1__   Day __2__   Date _____

Time	Meal Plans	Serving Size	(grams)
_____	**Breakfast**		
	Protein	2	
	Fruit or Grain	1½	
	Beverage	1	
_____	**Protein Snack**		
_____	**Lunch**		
	Protein	1½	
	Vegetable	1	
	Lettuce	Unl.	
	Fruit	1	
	Beverage	1	
	Miscellaneous	2	
_____	**Protein Snack**		
_____	**Dinner**		
	Protein	1½	
	Vegetable	1	
	Lettuce	Unl.	
	Fruit	1	
	Beverage	1	
	Miscellaneous	2	
_____	**Protein Snack**		
_____			
		TOTAL	

Weight _____

Vitamins   AM   Noon   PM

Fluids _____

Activities _____
_____
_____

Pedometer Steps _____

WEEKLY BODY MEASUREMENTS

Chest _____ Hips _____
Waist _____ Thighs _____
Abdomen _____

SUCCESS LEARNING TOOLS

Read pages # _____
Audio Tapes _____
Affirmation _____
_____
_____

Plan to Overcome Today's Obstacles:
_____
_____
_____
_____
_____
_____

Notes:
_____
_____
_____
_____

CHOOSE ONE DAY EACH WEEK DURING METABOLIC ADJUSTMENT
AS YOUR "PROTEIN DAY." DO YOUR "PROTEIN DAY" EXACTLY
AS YOU DID DURING WEIGHT LOSS.

Lean *for* Life®
DAILY ACTION PLAN

LEVEL I METABOLIC ADJUSTMENT

Week ___1___   Day ___3___   Date _____

Time	Meal Plans	Serving Size	(grams)
_____	**Breakfast**		
	Protein 2		
	Fruit or Grain 1½		
	Beverage 1		
_____	**Protein Snack**		
_____	**Lunch**		
	Protein 1½		
	Vegetable 1		
	Lettuce Unl.		
	Fruit 1		
	Beverage 1		
	Miscellaneous 2		
_____	**Protein Snack**		
_____	**Dinner**		
	Protein 1½		
	Vegetable 1		
	Lettuce Unl.		
	Fruit 1		
	Beverage 1		
	Miscellaneous 2		
_____	**Protein Snack**		
		TOTAL	

Weight _____

Vitamins   AM   Noon   PM

Fluids _____

Activities _____
_____
_____

Pedometer Steps _____

WEEKLY BODY MEASUREMENTS

Chest _____   Hips _____
Waist _____   Thighs _____
Abdomen _____

SUCCESS LEARNING TOOLS

Read pages # _____
Audio Tapes _____
Affirmation _____
_____

Plan to Overcome Today's Obstacles:
_____
_____
_____
_____
_____
_____
_____

Notes:
_____
_____
_____
_____

CHOOSE ONE DAY EACH WEEK DURING METABOLIC ADJUSTMENT AS YOUR "PROTEIN DAY." DO YOUR "PROTEIN DAY" EXACTLY AS YOU DID DURING WEIGHT LOSS.

Lean *for* Life®
DAILY ACTION PLAN

LEVEL 2 METABOLIC ADJUSTMENT

Week ____ **1** ____   Day ____ **4** ____   Date _____

Time	Meal Plans	Serving Size	(grams)
_____	**Breakfast**		
	Protein	2	
	Fruit or Grain	1½	
	Beverage	1	
_____	**Protein Snack**		
_____	**Lunch**		
	Protein	2	
	Vegetable	1	
	Lettuce	Unl.	
	Fruit	1	
	Beverage	1	
	Miscellaneous	2	
_____	**Protein Snack**		
_____	**Dinner**		
	Protein	2	
	Vegetable	1	
	Lettuce	Unl.	
	Fruit	1	
	Beverage	1	
	Miscellaneous	2	
_____	**Protein Snack**		
		TOTAL	

Weight _____

Vitamins   AM   Noon   PM

Fluids _____

Activities _____
_____
_____
_____

Pedometer Steps _____

WEEKLY BODY MEASUREMENTS

Chest _____   Hips _____
Waist _____   Thighs _____
Abdomen _____

SUCCESS LEARNING TOOLS

Read pages # _____
Audio Tapes _____
Affirmation _____
_____
_____

Plan to Overcome Today's Obstacles:
_____
_____
_____
_____
_____
_____
_____

Notes:
_____
_____
_____

CHOOSE ONE DAY EACH WEEK DURING METABOLIC ADJUSTMENT
AS YOUR "PROTEIN DAY." DO YOUR "PROTEIN DAY" EXACTLY
AS YOU DID DURING WEIGHT LOSS.

Lean *for* Life®
DAILY ACTION PLAN

LEVEL 2 METABOLIC ADJUSTMENT

Week __1__   Day __5__   Date _____

Time	Meal Plans	Serving Size	(grams)
_____	**Breakfast**		
	Protein	2	
	Fruit or Grain	1½	
	Beverage	1	
_____	**Protein Snack**		
_____	**Lunch**		
	Protein	2	
	Vegetable	1	
	Lettuce	Unl.	
	Fruit	1	
	Beverage	1	
	Miscellaneous	2	
_____	**Protein Snack**		
_____	**Dinner**		
	Protein	2	
	Vegetable	1	
	Lettuce	Unl.	
	Fruit	1	
	Beverage	1	
	Miscellaneous	2	
_____	**Protein Snack**		
		TOTAL	

Weight _____

Vitamins   AM   Noon   PM

Fluids _____

Activities _____
_____
_____

\# Pedometer Steps _____

WEEKLY BODY MEASUREMENTS

Chest _____   Hips _____
Waist _____   Thighs _____
Abdomen _____

SUCCESS LEARNING TOOLS

Read pages # _____
Audio Tapes _____
Affirmation _____
_____

Plan to Overcome Today's Obstacles:
_____
_____
_____
_____

Notes:
_____
_____
_____
_____

CHOOSE ONE DAY EACH WEEK DURING METABOLIC ADJUSTMENT AS YOUR "PROTEIN DAY." DO YOUR "PROTEIN DAY" EXACTLY AS YOU DID DURING WEIGHT LOSS.

Lean *for* Life®
DAILY ACTION PLAN

LEVEL 2 METABOLIC ADJUSTMENT

Week __I__   Day __6__   Date _____

Time	Meal Plans	Serving Size	(grams)
_____	**Breakfast**		
	Protein	2	
	Fruit or Grain	1½	
	Beverage	I	
_____	**Protein Snack**		
_____	**Lunch**		
	Protein	2	
	Vegetable	I	
	Lettuce	Unl.	
	Fruit	I	
	Beverage	I	
	Miscellaneous	2	
_____	**Protein Snack**		
_____	**Dinner**		
	Protein	2	
	Vegetable	I	
	Lettuce	Unl.	
	Fruit	I	
	Beverage	I	
	Miscellaneous	2	
_____	**Protein Snack**		
		TOTAL	

Weight _____

Vitamins   AM   Noon   PM

Fluids _____

Activities _____

_____

_____

Pedometer Steps _____

WEEKLY BODY MEASUREMENTS

Chest _____   Hips _____

Waist _____   Thighs _____

Abdomen _____

SUCCESS LEARNING TOOLS

Read pages # _____

Audio Tapes _____

Affirmation _____

_____

Plan to Overcome Today's Obstacles:

_____

_____

_____

_____

_____

Notes:

_____

_____

_____

_____

CHOOSE ONE DAY EACH WEEK DURING METABOLIC ADJUSTMENT AS YOUR "PROTEIN DAY." DO YOUR "PROTEIN DAY" EXACTLY AS YOU DID DURING WEIGHT LOSS.

Lean *for* Life®
DAILY ACTION PLAN

LEVEL 2 METABOLIC ADJUSTMENT

Week ___I___   Day ___7___   Date _____

Time	Meal Plans	Serving Size	(grams)
_____	**Breakfast**		
	Protein	2	
	Fruit or Grain	1½	
	Beverage	1	
_____	**Protein Snack**		
_____	**Lunch**		
	Protein	2	
	Vegetable	1	
	Lettuce	Unl.	
	Fruit	1	
	Beverage	1	
	Miscellaneous	2	
_____	**Protein Snack**		
_____	**Dinner**		
	Protein	2	
	Vegetable	1	
	Lettuce	Unl.	
	Fruit	1	
	Beverage	1	
	Miscellaneous	2	
_____	**Protein Snack**		
		TOTAL	

Weight _____
Vitamins   AM   Noon   PM
Fluids _____

Activities _____
_____
_____

Pedometer Steps _____

WEEKLY BODY MEASUREMENTS

Chest _____   Hips _____
Waist _____   Thighs _____
Abdomen _____

SUCCESS LEARNING TOOLS

Read pages # _____
Audio Tapes _____
Affirmation _____
_____

Plan to Overcome Today's Obstacles:
_____
_____
_____
_____
_____
_____

Notes:
_____
_____
_____
_____
_____

CHOOSE ONE DAY EACH WEEK DURING METABOLIC ADJUSTMENT
AS YOUR "PROTEIN DAY." DO YOUR "PROTEIN DAY" EXACTLY
AS YOU DID DURING WEIGHT LOSS.

Lean *for* Life®
DAILY ACTION PLAN

LEVEL 3 METABOLIC ADJUSTMENT

Week __2__   Day __8__   Date _____

Time	Meal Plans	Serving Size	(grams)
____	**Breakfast**		
	Protein	2	
	Fruit or Grain	1½	
	Beverage	1	
____	**Protein Snack**		
____	**Lunch**		
	Protein	2	
	Vegetable	1	
	Lettuce	Unl.	
	Fruit	1	
	Grain	1	
	Beverage	1	
	Miscellaneous	2	
____	**Protein Snack**		
____	**Dinner**		
	Protein	2	
	Vegetable	1	
	Lettuce	Unl.	
	Fruit	1	
	Grain	1	
	Beverage	1	
	Miscellaneous	2	
____	**Protein Snack**		
		TOTAL	

Weight _____

Vitamins   AM   Noon   PM

Fluids _____

Activities _____

Pedometer Steps _____

WEEKLY BODY MEASUREMENTS

Chest _____ Hips _____
Waist _____ Thighs _____
Abdomen _____

SUCCESS LEARNING TOOLS

Read pages # _____
Audio Tapes _____
Affirmation _____
_____
_____

Plan to Overcome Today's Obstacles:
_____
_____
_____
_____
_____
_____

Notes:
_____
_____
_____
_____

CHOOSE ONE DAY EACH WEEK DURING METABOLIC ADJUSTMENT
AS YOUR "PROTEIN DAY." DO YOUR "PROTEIN DAY" EXACTLY
AS YOU DID DURING WEIGHT LOSS.

Lean *for* Life®
DAILY ACTION PLAN

LEVEL 3 METABOLIC ADJUSTMENT

Week __2__ Day __9__ Date _____

Time	Meal Plans	Serving Size	(grams)
_____	**Breakfast**		
	Protein	2	
	Fruit or Grain	1½	
	Beverage	1	
_____	**Protein Snack**		
_____	**Lunch**		
	Protein	2	
	Vegetable	1	
	Lettuce	Unl.	
	Fruit	1	
	Grain	1	
	Beverage	1	
	Miscellaneous	2	
_____	**Protein Snack**		
_____	**Dinner**		
	Protein	2	
	Vegetable	1	
	Lettuce	Unl.	
	Fruit	1	
	Grain	1	
	Beverage	1	
	Miscellaneous	2	
_____	**Protein Snack**		
		TOTAL	

Weight _____

Vitamins   AM   Noon   PM

Fluids _____

Activities _____

_____

_____

\# Pedometer Steps _____

WEEKLY BODY MEASUREMENTS

Chest _____ Hips _____

Waist _____ Thighs _____

Abdomen _____

SUCCESS LEARNING TOOLS

Read pages # _____

Audio Tapes _____

Affirmation _____

_____

Plan to Overcome Today's Obstacles:

_____

_____

_____

_____

_____

_____

_____

Notes:

_____

_____

_____

_____

CHOOSE ONE DAY EACH WEEK DURING METABOLIC ADJUSTMENT AS YOUR "PROTEIN DAY." DO YOUR "PROTEIN DAY" EXACTLY AS YOU DID DURING WEIGHT LOSS.

Lean *for* Life®
DAILY ACTION PLAN

LEVEL 3 METABOLIC ADJUSTMENT

Week __2__   Day __10__   Date _____

Time	Meal Plans	Serving Size	(grams)
_____	**Breakfast**		
	Protein	2	
	Fruit or Grain	1½	
	Beverage	1	
_____	**Protein Snack**		
_____	**Lunch**		
	Protein	2	
	Vegetable	1	
	Lettuce	Unl.	
	Fruit	1	
	Grain	1	
	Beverage	1	
	Miscellaneous	2	
_____	**Protein Snack**		
_____	**Dinner**		
	Protein	2	
	Vegetable	1	
	Lettuce	Unl.	
	Fruit	1	
	Grain	1	
	Beverage	1	
	Miscellaneous	2	
_____	**Protein Snack**		
		TOTAL	

Weight _____

Vitamins   AM   Noon   PM

Fluids _____

Activities _____
_____
_____

\# Pedometer Steps _____

WEEKLY BODY MEASUREMENTS

Chest _____   Hips _____
Waist _____   Thighs _____
Abdomen _____

SUCCESS LEARNING TOOLS

Read pages # _____
Audio Tapes _____
Affirmation _____
_____

Plan to Overcome Today's Obstacles: _____
_____
_____
_____
_____
_____

Notes: _____
_____
_____
_____
_____

CHOOSE ONE DAY EACH WEEK DURING METABOLIC ADJUSTMENT AS YOUR "PROTEIN DAY." DO YOUR "PROTEIN DAY" EXACTLY AS YOU DID DURING WEIGHT LOSS.

Lean for Life®
DAILY ACTION PLAN

LEVEL 3 METABOLIC ADJUSTMENT

Week __2__ Day __11__ Date _____

Time	Meal Plans		Serving Size	(grams)
	Breakfast			
	Protein	2		
	Fruit or Grain	1½		
	Beverage	1		
	Protein Snack			
	Lunch			
	Protein	2		
	Vegetable	1		
	Lettuce	Unl.		
	Fruit	1		
	Grain	1		
	Beverage	1		
	Miscellaneous	2		
	Protein Snack			
	Dinner			
	Protein	2		
	Vegetable	1		
	Lettuce	Unl.		
	Fruit	1		
	Grain	1		
	Beverage	1		
	Miscellaneous	2		
	Protein Snack			
			TOTAL	

Weight _____

Vitamins   AM   Noon   PM

Fluids _____

Activities _____

Pedometer Steps _____

WEEKLY BODY MEASUREMENTS

Chest _____   Hips _____

Waist _____   Thighs _____

Abdomen _____

SUCCESS LEARNING TOOLS

Read pages # _____

Audio Tapes _____

Affirmation _____

Plan to Overcome Today's Obstacles:

Notes:

CHOOSE ONE DAY EACH WEEK DURING METABOLIC ADJUSTMENT AS YOUR "PROTEIN DAY." DO YOUR "PROTEIN DAY" EXACTLY AS YOU DID DURING WEIGHT LOSS.

Lean *for* Life®
DAILY ACTION PLAN

LEVEL 3 METABOLIC ADJUSTMENT

Week __2__   Day __12__   Date _____

Time	Meal Plans	Serving Size	(grams)
_____	**Breakfast**		
	Protein	2	
	Fruit or Grain	1½	
	Beverage	1	
_____	**Protein Snack**		
_____	**Lunch**		
	Protein	2	
	Vegetable	1	
	Lettuce	Unl.	
	Fruit	1	
	Grain	1	
	Beverage	1	
	Miscellaneous	2	
_____	**Protein Snack**		
_____	**Dinner**		
	Protein	2	
	Vegetable	1	
	Lettuce	Unl.	
	Fruit	1	
	Grain	1	
	Beverage	1	
	Miscellaneous	2	
_____	**Protein Snack**		
		TOTAL	

Weight _____

Vitamins ___ AM ___ Noon ___ PM

Fluids _____

Activities _____

\# Pedometer Steps _____

WEEKLY BODY MEASUREMENTS

Chest _____   Hips _____

Waist _____   Thighs _____

Abdomen _____

SUCCESS LEARNING TOOLS

Read pages # _____

Audio Tapes _____

Affirmation _____

Plan to Overcome Today's Obstacles:
_____
_____
_____
_____
_____
_____

Notes:
_____
_____
_____
_____

CHOOSE ONE DAY EACH WEEK DURING METABOLIC ADJUSTMENT AS YOUR "PROTEIN DAY." DO YOUR "PROTEIN DAY" EXACTLY AS YOU DID DURING WEIGHT LOSS.

Lean *for* Life®
DAILY ACTION PLAN

LEVEL 3 METABOLIC ADJUSTMENT

Week ___2___   Day ___13___   Date _____

Time	Meal Plans	Serving Size	(grams)
_____	**Breakfast**		
	Protein	2	
	Fruit or Grain	1½	
	Beverage	1	
_____	**Protein Snack**		
_____	**Lunch**		
	Protein	2	
	Vegetable	1	
	Lettuce	Unl.	
	Fruit	1	
	Grain	1	
	Beverage	1	
	Miscellaneous	2	
_____	**Protein Snack**		
_____	**Dinner**		
	Protein	2	
	Vegetable	1	
	Lettuce	Unl.	
	Fruit	1	
	Grain	1	
	Beverage	1	
	Miscellaneous	2	
_____	**Protein Snack**		
		TOTAL	

Weight _____
Vitamins   AM ____ Noon ____ PM ____
Fluids _____

Activities _____
_____
_____

Pedometer Steps _____

WEEKLY BODY MEASUREMENTS

Chest _____   Hips _____
Waist _____   Thighs _____
Abdomen _____

SUCCESS LEARNING TOOLS

Read pages # _____
Audio Tapes _____
Affirmation _____
_____

Plan to Overcome Today's Obstacles:
_____
_____
_____
_____
_____
_____

Notes:
_____
_____
_____
_____

CHOOSE ONE DAY EACH WEEK DURING METABOLIC ADJUSTMENT AS YOUR "PROTEIN DAY." DO YOUR "PROTEIN DAY" EXACTLY AS YOU DID DURING WEIGHT LOSS.

Lean *for* Life®
DAILY ACTION PLAN

LEVEL 3 METABOLIC ADJUSTMENT

Week __2__   Day __14__   Date _____

Time	Meal Plans	Serving Size	(grams)
_____	**Breakfast**		
	Protein	2	
	Fruit or Grain	1½	
	Beverage	1	
_____	**Protein Snack**		
_____	**Lunch**		
	Protein	2	
	Vegetable	1	
	Lettuce	Unl.	
	Fruit	1	
	Grain	1	
	Beverage	1	
	Miscellaneous	2	
_____	**Protein Snack**		
_____	**Dinner**		
	Protein	2	
	Vegetable	1	
	Lettuce	Unl.	
	Fruit	1	
	Grain	1	
	Beverage	1	
	Miscellaneous	2	
_____	**Protein Snack**		
		TOTAL	

Weight _____

Vitamins   AM   Noon   PM

Fluids _____

Activities _____

_____

_____

\# Pedometer Steps _____

WEEKLY BODY MEASUREMENTS

Chest _____ Hips _____

Waist _____ Thighs _____

Abdomen _____

SUCCESS LEARNING TOOLS

Read pages # _____

Audio Tapes _____

Affirmation _____

_____

Plan to Overcome Today's Obstacles:

_____

_____

_____

_____

_____

_____

Notes: _____

_____

_____

_____

CHOOSE ONE DAY EACH WEEK DURING METABOLIC ADJUSTMENT AS YOUR "PROTEIN DAY." DO YOUR "PROTEIN DAY" EXACTLY AS YOU DID DURING WEIGHT LOSS.

PHASE 2: LIFETIME MAINTENANCE

You'll discover how to stabilize at your new lean weight so you can eat normally without regaining weight

Today's Eating Plan

If you have achieved your lean weight goal, you're ready to begin Phase 2: Lifetime Maintenance. If, however, you have more weight to lose, you'll return to Phase 1: Weight Loss today and repeat another cycle.

Imagine, if you will, a weight loss program called "The Amazing Yo-Yo Diet." On it, you would lose all the weight you wanted. You would look terrific and feel fabulous. People would compliment you on your success.

Then, within days of achieving your goal, you would gradually begin regaining the weight—a pound here, a half-pound there. Over time, the sense of pride and accomplishment you initially felt would be eclipsed by disappointment and disbelief as you realized you had gained back every single pound you'd lost.

Sounds more like an exercise in frustration and futility than an effective approach to weight loss, doesn't it? Yet that's exactly what millions of people do every year. Studies show that more than 95% of those who complete weight loss programs regain their weight within five years. Why? Because instead of embracing their success by learning how to maintain their lean weight, they revert back to the habits that made them fat in the first place. By committing to *losing* weight but not to *keeping it off,* they win the battle but lose the war.

It doesn't have to be that way. This program is called Lean for Life for good reason. It not only helps you lose weight, it shows you how you can maintain your new lean weight for life! Follow the Lean for Life program through "Phase 2: Lifetime Maintenance" and you'll never need to diet again.

THE CHALLENGE

Lifetime Maintenance is more than a phase of a weight control program. It's a mindset and an attitude. It's about taking care of yourself and making healthy choices. It's an on-going, day-by-day process of recommitting yourself to the excellence you've achieved. During the first three to six months of "Phase 2: Lifetime Maintenance," you will gradually add a variety of foods to your diet to determine how much your body can tolerate without a weight gain, all while continuing to practice the success strategies you learned during the Weight Loss phase of the program.

Many people find "Phase 2: Lifetime Maintenance" to be the most challenging part of the program. Some don't fully appreciate the value and benefits of this final phase. Their "urgency factor" is no longer quite so urgent. And since they're feeling healthier and more attractive, the need to do the work necessary to maintain often doesn't seem as pressing as their need to lose weight did just weeks earlier. On the heels of their recent success, it's easy to persuade themselves they've been "cured"—that they've "done it" and are finally "over the hump." Unfortunately, the value of—and the need for—"Phase 2: Lifetime Maintenance" often doesn't become apparent until it's too late.

If you want to maintain your weight loss, you must maintain the behavior changes that made it happen. That's exactly what "Phase 2: Lifetime Maintenance" is designed to help you do. Like Phase 1: Weight Loss, it has been revised, refined, and perfected over more than 30 years. It works! Thousands of Lindora patients who have lost weight on other programs, only to gain it all back, have successfully maintained their weight loss by practicing the basic principles of this second phase. You can, too.

STABILIZING AT YOUR NEW LEAN WEIGHT

During "Phase 2: Lifetime Maintenance," your goal is simple and specific—to stabilize at your new lean weight so that you will be able to eat normally without gaining weight. This is a crucial step because even after you've reached your lean weight, your body's setpoint remains elevated. If you begin eating the way you have in the past, you will very likely regain the weight just as rapidly as you lost it.

In order to stabilize your body at your new lean weight, it's critical that you maintain your weight within three pounds long enough to allow the weight-regulating center in your hypothalamus to accept your

DR. STAMPER

"During Lifetime Maintenance, it's important to continue doing those things that helped you *become* Lean for Life."

"There are plenty of alibis for failure. Success doesn't need them."

— Anonymous

new weight as "normal" and to make adjustments in the metabolic feedback system we discussed back on Day 4. This, in turn, helps to reset your setpoint.

Remember when we likened the setpoint to a thermostat? When you're overweight, your setpoint adjusts upward to accommodate your body's increased caloric needs. When you lose weight, you need to adjust your setpoint downward so that it doesn't set off those annoying metabolic "alarm bells"—the ones that lead to cravings, urges to overeat, overeating, weight gain, and that maddening cycle known as "yo-yo dieting."

ACHIEVING EQUILIBRIUM

The process of resetting your setpoint and stabilizing your weight typically takes at least three to twelve months. After three months, you can determine whether you've stabilized at your new weight and reached equilibrium. Equilibrium is a state in which your weight has stabilized and your setpoint has readjusted, making it possible for you to eat more while still maintaining your lean weight.

How will you know whether you've achieved equilibrium? By eating a "test meal," a large evening meal of balanced food groups that is larger than you are accustomed to eating. How much larger depends on how much you're currently eating. A 200-pound man, for example, can eat—and therefore add—more food than a 100-pound woman. If your body has reached equilibrium at its new lean weight, your weight will stay approximately the same, even after your "test meal."

If you do gain, you'll know your body has not yet stabilized at its new weight. If this happens, you'll need to get back to your lean weight by having only protein for your evening meals until you lose the weight you've regained. Once you've done that, your goal then becomes to stay within three pounds of your lean weight for another three to four weeks. Then try again with another test meal until you can eat it without gaining weight.

Once your body has stabilized at its lean weight, you'll find you can eat more food—within reason—and not gain weight. But because your body may always be sensitive to large quantities of carbohydrates and fats, you most likely won't be able to resume your old eating habits without a weight gain. You will, however, be able to eat generous amounts of healthy foods—and occasionally even splurge—and still stay Lean for Life.

LEAN FOODS VS. FAT FOODS

At Lindora, we encourage patients beginning "Phase 2: Lifetime Maintenance" to think of foods in two categories: Lean Foods and Fat Foods.

WHAT STRESS CAN DO TO YOUR BODY AND YOUR BRAIN

It's no secret that stress takes its toll on the human body. It can cause a variety of health problems ranging from hives and headaches to severe muscle tension, stomach disorders, and even weight gain.

Some experts are more convinced than ever that sustained stress can also wreak havoc on—and in—your brain, too. A study published in *Science* magazine reports that brain scans (MRI's) performed on people who have endured long-term stress during combat or childhood abuse show a significant decrease in the size of certain parts of their brains, providing compelling evidence of the connection between our minds and bodies.

So make a point to continue practicing your stress management skills. They'll not only ease the pressure and help you stay Lean for Life, but your brain will be healthier, too!

Lean foods contain less than 30% fat calories and are low or moderate in simple carbohydrates. These foods—especially those with less than 15% fat calories—are the foundation for maintaining your new lean weight. Lean foods also include fruits, vegetables, and grains prepared with no (or very low) amounts of fat and sugar.

Foods with 20% to 30% fat calories are to be eaten as tolerated. This means that as you begin reintroducing these higher fat foods—and especially higher carbohydrate foods—into your daily diet, you'll need to pay close attention to how your body metabolizes them. If you find you're gradually gaining weight, you'll know that you're sensitive to these foods and must eat them less often.

Fat foods contain more than 30% fat calories. Foods that are high in calories from carbs or fat and low in nutritional value also fall into this category. Eat too much "fat food" such as candy, cookies, junk food, and fast food, and you will gain weight. If you're not careful, you can easily consume more calories in a single meal of fat foods than your body needs for an entire day. Review the section on how to read food labels on page 194.

If you do choose to eat fat foods, be aware of how much and how often you're eating them. Set limits. Remember that the fat you eat is the fat you wear. Eating well—and staying Lean for Life—is a choice you will need to make every day. Ultimately, how you eat, what you eat, and when you eat is up to you. The choice is always yours.

"SO WHAT DO I EAT?"

Over the next three to 12 months, you'll follow the same basic meal structure as you did during Metabolic Adjustment, but with one major difference—you'll enjoy more choices. In addition to the food choices in Phase 1, you'll be able to eat a variety of other healthy foods. Your Menu Plan will include:

PROTEINS
3 daily servings (one per meal)

Your choice of one serving (average 100-200 calories each) at breakfast, lunch, and dinner. Be sure to weigh meat, seafood, and poultry after removing any skin, bone, and visible fat. Broil, boil, barbecue, microwave, roast, or "fry" using Pam spray or an equivalent. Your healthiest choices are high-protein foods that are lowest in fat and calories. Read labels on canned or packaged proteins carefully.

VEGETABLES
At least two daily servings

Choose at least two servings (average 40 calories each) a day, one each at lunch and dinner. Lettuce and other leafy greens? Have all you want. Measure vegetables raw, frozen (thawed), or water packed (drained). Read labels on packaged food for exact calories.

GRAINS
3 servings (men may tolerate more)

Choose three servings a day (average 100 calories each) of whole grain bread, rice, pasta, crackers, and cereals, as tolerated. This simply means that if you find yourself regaining weight, eliminate one grain serving. Remember that grains are high in carbohydrates, so choose accordingly. Limit dry cereals to one cup and cooked cereals to 3/4 cup per serving. Note that the percentage of fat in snack crackers varies between 30% to 50% or more. Choose low-fat or nonfat crackers that don't exceed 30% fat.

FRUITS
3 daily servings (one per meal)

Your choice of three servings (average 90 calories each), incuding at least one citrus fruit every day. Choose fresh, frozen (thawed), or water packed, with no sugar or juice added.

FAT
3 servings

Choose three servings a day (average 100 calories each). Remember that fat has nine calories per gram—more than double the number of calories per gram of carbohydrates or protein. Be sure to limit your fat calories to no more than 30%. Again, read labels carefully—while Fat

Free Promise Ultra Light and Fleischmann's Non-Fat Margarine have just five calories per serving, most other "diet" and "light" margarines are 100% calories from fat. Since most foods contain some fat, you need to pay close attention to what you're eating to make sure that fat doesn't "sneak" into your diet and back on to your body. Before you eat it, ask yourself, "Is it worth it?"

SNACKS
3 protein choices per day

Continue the habit of mid-morning, mid-afternoon, and evening snacks—and continue to make them proteins!

MISCELLANEOUS
Unlimited

Be sure to count the calories of all miscellaneous foods. Miscellaneous foods include any items that are five calories per serving or less.

DESSERT
(Optional: One daily serving; counts as a grain or fruit serving)

Dessert? In a "diet book"? That's right! Now that you've gotten down to your lean weight, you have choices that wouldn't have been productive during Weight Loss. One of them is the option of having a four-ounce serving of fat-free ice cream or frozen yogurt containing 90 calories or less as a substitution for one of your daily fruit or grain servings. You can also try low-fat ice cream, but steer clear of any that have more than 30% fat or more than 100 calories per four-ounce serving.

Notice that all your meals are based on protein, just as they were during the Weight Loss phase of the program. Be sure to eat all your protein servings to avoid becoming hungry and to help control cravings. Now that you've achieved your lean weight, there's more flexibility in your plan as to what you eat and when you eat it. If, for example, you have two grain servings at lunch and none at dinner, it's not going to affect your weight. But if you start having two at lunch and one or two at dinner, you'll probably begin noticing a gradual weight increase. Watch out for this. Also be sure to start your day with a healthy breakfast. Breakfast-skippers invariably end up becoming night-time snackers and weight-gainers.

It's a good idea to buy a food content book—they're available in paperback—that lists the calories, protein, carbohydrate, and fat content in thousands of foods. Remember that you'll no longer be counting carbohydrates for ketosis. You will, however, want to keep close tabs on how much you're eating and the carbs, protein, and fat it contains.

"HOW MUCH CAN I EAT?"

WOMEN

ACTIVE (6,000 steps or more per day on pedometer)
12-14 calories per pound of body weight

Weight	Calories per day	Carbohydrates - 45% 1 gram = 4 cal Calories / grams	Protein - 25% 1 gram = 4 cal Calories / grams	Fat - 30% or less 1 gram = 9 cal Calories / grams
100 lb.	1,200-1,400	540-630 / 135-158	300-350 / 75-88	360-420 / 40-47
120 lb.	1,440-1,680	648-756 / 162-189	360-420 / 90-105	432-504 / 48-56
140 lb.	1,680-1,960	756-882 / 189-221	420-490 / 105-123	504-588 / 56-65
160 lb.	1,920-2,240	864-1,008 / 216-252	480-560 / 120-140	576-672 / 64-75

INACTIVE (5,000 steps or less per day on pedometer)
10-12 calories per pound of body weight

Weight	Calories per day	Carbohydrates - 45% 1 gram = 4 cal Calories / grams	Protein - 25% 1 gram = 4 cal Calories / grams	Fat - 30% or less 1 gram = 9 cal Calories / grams
100 lb.	1,000-1,200	450-540 / 113-135	250-300 / 63-75	300-360 / 33-40
120 lb.	1,200-1,440	540-648 / 135-162	300-360 / 75-90	360-432 / 40-48
140 lb.	1,400-1,680	630-756 / 158-189	350-420 / 88-105	420-504 / 47-56
160 lb.	1,600-1,920	720-864 / 180-216	400-480 / 100-120	480-576 / 53-64

MEN

ACTIVE (6,000 steps or more per day on pedometer)
14-16 calories per pound of body weight

Weight	Calories per day	Carbohydrates - 45% 1 gram = 4 cal Calories / grams	Protein - 25% 1 gram = 4 cal Calories / grams	Fat - 30% or less 1 gram = 9 cal Calories / grams
150 lb.	2,100-2,400	945-1,080 / 236-270	525-600 / 131-150	630-720 / 70-80
170 lb.	2,380-2,720	1,071-1,224 / 268-306	595-680 / 149-170	714-816 / 79-91
190 lb.	2,660-3,040	1,197-1,368 / 299-342	665-760 / 166-190	798-912 / 89-101
210 lb.	2,940-3,360	1,323-1,512 / 331-378	735-840 / 184-210	882-1,008 / 98-112

INACTIVE (5,000 steps or less per day on pedometer)
12-14 calories per pound of body weight

Weight	Calories per day	Carbohydrates - 45% 1 gram = 4 cal Calories / grams	Protein - 25% 1 gram = 4 cal Calories / grams	Fat - 30% or less 1 gram = 9 cal Calories / grams
150 lb.	1,800-2,100	810-945 / 203-236	450-525 / 113-131	540-630 / 60-70
170 lb.	2,040-2,380	918-1,071 / 230-268	510-595 / 128-149	612-714 / 68-79
190 lb.	2,280-2,660	1,026-1,197 / 257-299	570-665 / 143-166	684-798 / 76-89
210 lb.	2,520-2,940	1,134-1,323 / 284-331	630-735 / 158-184	756-882 / 84-98

FAT-BUSTERS: EASY WAYS TO REDUCE YOUR FAT INTAKE

❑ Bake, braise, broil, roast, barbecue, or microwave all meats, fish and poultry. "Stir fry" or sauté in fat free broth. No frying.

❑ Steam vegetables in a little water, then add herbs and lemon instead of butter.

❑ Choose nonfat margarines and spreads. There are a number of new ones on the market.

❑ Choose whole grain breads and pasta instead of those made with refined white flour.

❑ Limit your consumption of red meats. Choose turkey breast, chicken, and fish.

❑ Trim all visible fat and skin from meats and poultry.

❑ Make salad dressings from nonfat yogurt and nonfat mayonnaise. Try bottled nonfat, low-calorie dressings.

❑ Substitute nonfat or low-fat cheese for the high-fat, high-calorie variety.

❑ Stir-fry fresh vegetables in bouillon or fat free broth.

o Read labels carefully to determine how many of the calories are from fat. Choose accordingly.

"HOW MUCH CAN I EAT?"

How much food you'll be able to eat without gaining weight depends on a number of factors, including your gender, current weight, and level of activity.

An inactive 140-pound woman, for example, typically needs only 10 to 12 calories per pound of body weight to maintain her weight—somewhere in the neighborhood of 1,400 to 1,680 calories. An active 190-pound man, on the other hand, may be able to consume 14 to 16 calories per pound of body weight—2,660 and 3,040 calories—without gaining weight.

The chart on the previous page will help you estimate how many calories your body needs to maintain your present weight. It will also help you plan meals to ensure that you achieve a healthy balance of 45% carbohydrates, 25% protein, and 30% or less in fat. What's more, it helps you easily estimate how many grams of protein, carbohydrates, and fat you need.

DR. STAMPER

"The strategies that helped you succeed in losing weight will also help you maintain your weight."

To maximize your results, restrict your fat grams even more—35 to 45 grams for women, and 45 to 60 grams for men. The calories you "save" can then be used for either more protein or more healthy complex carbohydrates. Over time, you'll learn what works best for you. If you find yourself feeling hungry and rummaging through the cupboards for food when you know you've eaten enough, take a good look at what you've eaten during the day. You'll probably discover that you've eaten too many carbohydrates and not enough protein. As you know, eating protein will fill you up and satisfy your hunger, while eating carbohydrates will usually stimulate cravings and cause you to feel hungry. Each person is unique. Learn how your body reacts—and plan your food choices accordingly.

SUCCESS STRATEGIES: 10 WAYS TO GUARANTEE RESULTS DURING "PHASE 2: LIFETIME MAINTENANCE"

Want to continue enjoying the benefits of being Lean for Life? Keep doing those things that helped you accomplish your weight loss goal and you will!

1. *Maintain a support system.* This is especially important during the first twelve months of "Phase 2: Lifetime Maintenance." Whether you get support from friends, family members, at one of our clinics, or through the Lean for Life site on the World Wide Web, make a point to stay connected with people who appreciate what you've accomplished.

2. *Continue your moderate exercise.* This, too, must become a lifetime habit. Not only will exercise help you maintain your lean weight, but it also helps you control your appetite.

3. *Continue maintaining your Daily Action Plan until your weight has stabilized.* Behavior researchers report that people who are most successful at keeping their weight off are those who maintain a written record of their food and exercise. Whenever you find yourself regaining weight, keep a Daily Action Plan. It will help you regain awareness and regain control.

4. *Continue to weigh yourself every morning.* Make morning weigh-ins a lifetime habit. Addressing a minor weight gain today is much easier than being "surprised" by a 20-pound increase six months from now. Many successful maintainers tape their lean weight to their scale as a reminder. If you gain more than three pounds from your lean weight at any time during the first three to twelve months of "Phase 2: Lifetime Maintenance," have only protein for dinner

until you've returned to your lean weight. Once you've stabilized your weight, do a Protein Day any time you gain more than three pounds. Take charge of the situation.

5. ***Continue eating three meals a day.*** This important pattern helps to program your mind and body when to eat. If you start eating whenever you decide you're "hungry" or whenever you "have time," odds are you'll end up snacking on whatever is handy rather than planning a healthy meal. When you do snack, think protein, fruits, and vegetables. Steer clear of high-carbohydrate snacks. Carbs can make you hungry if your body has difficulty metabolizing them.

6. ***Continue doing one "Protein Day" every week.*** This will help you maintain a sense of awareness and control over your eating, and will also help curb your appetite. Many successful maintainers choose Monday as their "Protein Day." This keeps them focused and in control as they begin each week. Some Lindora patients who have maintained their lean weight for more than 10 years find that when they begin each week with a full Protein Day or a protein breakfast and lunch—and then have a sensible dinner that evening—they can more easily control their appetite throughout the rest of the week.

7. ***Continue drinking at least 80 ounces of calorie-free liquid every day.*** This cleanses your system, helps curb appetite, and reduces fluid retention.

8. ***Continue taking vitamins.*** While you're probably eating healthier now than you ever have, taking a high quality multi-vitamin and mineral supplement every day helps insure that your body gets everything it needs to operate at peak efficiency.

9. ***Continue to watch your caffeine and alcohol consumption.*** Both can stimulate appetite—and alcohol contains empty calories. One shot of hard liquor totals around 100 calories.

10. ***Continue doing your mental training exercises.*** Mental training techniques such as affirmations, brief visualizations, and Daily Mental Training sessions help focus your attention, adjust your energy level, and increase your confidence. These important tools helped get you where you are. They can also help you maintain your success.

"Life is a mirror and will reflect back to the thinker what he thinks into it."

— Ernest Holmes

THE 4 HABITS OF HIGHLY SUCCESSFUL MAINTAINERS

Why do some people succeed while others stumble? Over the years, the medical staff at Lindora has observed that virtually all successful maintainers exhibit four "habits" that clearly contribute to their success:

1. ***Successful maintainers continue to practice the basics of the program.*** You've just spent the past six weeks or more learning the basics and learning how to make them work for you. They helped get you this far—why would you abandon them now? On page 248, you'll find a list of 10 success strategies. Put them into action and you'll continue to be successful, too.

2. ***Successful maintainers intentionally develop and maintain their self-image as a lean person.*** How can you do the same? By making positive affirmations a part of your everyday life. By visualizing yourself as a thin person. By practicing an "achievement attitude" of optimism and positive problem-solving. You can use mental training techniques to experience yourself in particular situations, looking and feeling successful at your lean weight. You can avoid old patterns of overeating and inactivity.

3. ***Successful maintainers are physically active.*** How active do you need to be? Some people can maintain their weight by walking 30 minutes a day, while others need to walk more. The only way to determine how much activity is enough is to keep track of your exercise and see how it affects your weight. If you find that you're gaining weight even when you average 30 minutes of moderate exercise a day, see what happens if you increase it to 45 minutes. If your weight creeps up when you average 10,000 steps a day on your step counter, see what happens if you average 12,000 steps a day. Resolve to do whatever it takes. And remember, walking isn't your only option. As long as it's moderate, you can ride a bike, dance, swim, do water aerobics, in-line skate, ski, or use a variety of exercise machines at your local gym. One of the great benefits of becoming Lean for Life is that you've transformed yourself into an active person. Except for quitting smoking, this is the single most positive step a person can take to ensure lifetime good health.

4. ***Successful maintainers plan ahead for high-risk situations.*** You and you alone are responsible for the choices you make. You can support yourself by anticipating challenges and developing a plan of action for managing potentially difficult situations. What will you do when a co-worker shows up with a platter of homemade brownies? When a snowstorm keeps you from walking outdoors?

Your Turn

Take time to revisit the MENTORS Daily Mental Training exercise from Day 16 (page 157). It can help you focus on:

❑ resetting your setpoint to your new, leaner weight

❑ seeing yourself making healthy, appropriate food choices

❑ enjoying feeling enthused and energized while exercising

❑ increasing the strength and flexibility of your muscles

These tapes can be even more beneficial during Lifetime Maintenance. This type of mental training has been proven to be extremely effective. Did you know that nearly 100% of the athletes competing in the 1996 Summer Olympics engaged in some form of mental training? Let these proven techniques help you achieve your own "gold medal" in your quest to become— and stay—Lean for Life!

Food for Thought

"Go confidently in the direction of your dreams. Live the life you have imagined."

— Henry David Thoreau

When you think ahead, you think more clearly—and react more effectively.

YOUR FUTURE—AND WELCOME TO IT!

Lifetime maintenance is clearly a journey rather than a destination. To paraphrase Anne Kaiser Stearns, whose wise words appear on the first page of this book, "If you keep doing what you've been doing, you'll keep getting the results you've gotten."

And if you don't, you won't. Any successful long-term maintainer will tell you that maintaining his or her lean weight requires determination, dedication, and discipline.

Your journey isn't over. If you've just completed Metabolic Adjustment and are moving on to Phase 2: Lifetime Maintenance, you've certainly ended a very positive part of your journey. Yet no matter how successful you've been in achieving your Lean for Life weight goal, remember that *maintaining* your result is ultimately what matters. I'd like to invite you to continue your journey to a lifetime of health with our *Lean for Life Phase 2: Lifetime Solutions* book, which guides you day-by-day through the challenges—and rewards—of weight maintenance. Along the way, you'll gain knowledge and develop vital, valuable skills that will help you stay focused and committed to new, healthful behaviors.

A year from now, where will you be in your journey? Will *you* be a Lean for life success story?

The choice, as always, is yours.

Lean *for* Life

RESOURCES

A Message to Your Doctor

Your personal physician can be a valuable resource as you

do the Lean for Life program. We encourage you to

photocopy the following page from the book and give it

to your doctor so that he or she can easily contact Lindora's

executive medical director for additional information.

Dear Doctor:

As a physician who has dedicated his career to the treatment of obesity and its co-morbid medical conditions for more than twenty years, I understand how challenging the treatment of obesity can be.

I believe the scientifically sound, common sense approach of the Lean for Life program offers new hope and a strong, supportive structure to those people who desperately want—and need—to lose weight. This book is intended to be a therapeutic tool and treatment adjunct, to be used with your guidance to help your patient safely lose excess weight—and keep it off for life.

While *Lean for Life Phase One: Weight Loss* provides your patient with a solid working knowledge of the science of fat loss, we at Lindora know that you—the physician who best knows the patient—are in a position to be his or her most valuable resource. There are a number of medications and medication combinations, for example, that may be appropriate adjunctive treatment for some patients, yet only after a professional assessment can such decisions be made. We have extensive experience with the use of medications and different prescription protocols that have proven to be effective.

I welcome the opportunity to be of service to you and your patients. If you would like to consult with me or receive more information on a medically supervised version of the Lean for Life program, please call or write to me at:

Lindora, Inc.
3505 Cadillac Avenue, Suite N-2
Costa Mesa, CA 92626
714/979-5680x253

Sincerely,

Peter D. Vash, M.D., M.P.H.

Peter D. Vash, M.D., M.P.H.
Executive Medical Director, Lindora, Inc.
Assistant Clinical Professor, UCLA School of Medicine
Past President, American Society of Bariatric Physicians

SERVICES

ORIGINAL MEDICALLY SUPERVISED PROGRAM

The Lindora clinic system is the largest medical organization in the United States specializing in the treatment of obesity and overweight. For information on the Lean for Life clinical program, to book a free consultation, or to learn the address of a clinic near you, call 1-888-LINDORA.

Lindora
COMPREHENSIVE MEDICAL WEIGHT CONTROL

Lean for Life® atWork

Enjoy the benefits of a weight control program in the convenience of your workplace. Health care providers such as HealthNet, Blue Cross of California, and UNICARE offer special discounts on Lean for Life programs and products. For more information regarding the "atWork" program, have your human resources or corporate wellness professional call 1-888-LINDORA.

LEAN FOR LIFE atHOME "atHome But Not Alone™"

Telecoaching

If you have a telephone, you have the basic tool needed to lose weight and learn to keep it off. The At Home But Not Alone™ program combines the clinically tested weight loss program with a personal coach to guide, support, and inform you. For more information, call **1-888-LINDORA**.

Internet

Visit our web site at **www.leanforlife.com** 24 hours a day, 7 days a week, and access the latest information on weight management, learn all about Lindora and the Lean for Life programs, e-mail your questions to our experts, participate in forums, order products and chat with others who, like you, are learning to be lean for life.

Lean for Life® Online

Lean for Life® Online is a personalized daily weight management system that delivers a level of support, information, and personal accountability you won't find anywhere else online. The interactive 45-day Lean for Life Online program includes:

- live access to Lindora program experts
- personalized charts and graphs that change daily to reflect your progress
- a convenient "To Do Today" list to guide you through your program
- daily audio and e-mail messages to help keep you focused and motivated
- unlimited access to our exclusive WebPal support system
- "Ask Debbie," "Motivation Central," and expert answers to questions
- special discounts on Lindora products
- a "StartSmart" kit featuring a copy of *Lean for Life Phase One: Weight Loss* and a variety pack of delicious Lean for Life high-protein nutrition bars, a Lean for Life Activity Monitor, Fat Burning Indicators (ketone sticks), and a "Getting Started" audio tape

For more information on Lean for Life Online, go to **www.leanforlife.com** or call **1-888-LINDORA.**

PRODUCTS

EAT BETTER

LEAN FOR LIFE
HIGH PROTEIN NUTRITION PRODUCTS

Bars • Soups • Shakes • Puddings • Drinks • Hot Dishes

- Clinically proven to enhance weight loss and weight maintenance
- High in bio-available protein
- Low in carbohydrates
- Specifically formulated to help control cravings and maintain weight
- Convenient and Delicious

RECIPE BOOK

Recipes for everyday and for special occasions, the *Lean for Life Recipe Book* is filled with simple, delicious recipes, including many featuring delicious Lean for Life products.

VITAMINS

These high-quality nutritional supplements are packed with vitamins and minerals and are specially formulated to enhance the Lean for Life program.

KETONE STRIPS

With these Fat Burning Indicators, you'll know immediately if you're burning fat! (For use during weight loss programs.)

MOVE MORE

STEP COUNTER

The Lean for Life Pedometer is light, attractive, and fun to wear. A great way to be sure that you're getting the exercise you need and the results you want.

STRESS LESS

A U D I O   T A P E S

LEAN FOR LIFE Tape Series

This set of five informative, motivational audio cassette tapes includes "Getting Started: The Six Essentials," "Identifying and Eliminating Defensive Barriers," "Relaxation and Guided Visualization," "Affirmations," and "Compulsive Cravings."

MENTORS™ Daily Mental Training Audio Cassette Tapes
Herman M. Frankel, M.D. and Jean Staeheli of Portland Health Institute

As nationally prominent experts in the field of mental training, Herman M. Frankel, M.D. and Jean Staeheli work together conducting clinical programs and research at Portland Health Institute. Their tapes are designed to support you in making positive structural changes in your body and your brain.

Basic MENTORS™ Program

1. My Peaceful Place
2. Enjoying My Food Choices
3. Enjoying my Physical Activity
4. Returning To The Path

Advanced MENTORS™ Program

5. Letting Go of What I No Longer Need
6. The Keeper of the Garden of Roses
7. The Child in the Chamber in the Castle
8. The Traveler and the Journey
9. My Healing Place

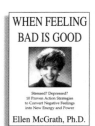

WHEN FEELING BAD IS GOOD: The Action Strategies
Spend an hour with Dr. Ellen McGrath

In this empowering 60-minute audio cassette tape, Dr. McGrath shares with you the best of what she has learned during her 28-year practice as a clinical psychologist. ACTION—not just talking and thinking—is the critical step in successfully maintaining weight loss.

BOOKS

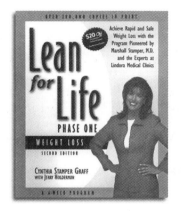

LEAN FOR LIFE PHASE ONE: WEIGHT LOSS
by Cynthia Stamper Graff
with Jerry Holderman

Lean for Life Phase One: Weight Loss is more than a book you read. It's a book you do! Whether you choose to lose five, 50, or 500 pounds, you'll find this remarkable, results-oriented book—and the clinically proven program it features—a dynamic roadmap to results. This innovative two-phase approach to weight loss has changed the lives and bodies of more than 200,000 men, women, and teens since 1971. It guides you through the program day by day, offering practical, proven "success strategies" and sharing inspiring insights from people who have lost between 20 and 450 pounds —and kept it off!

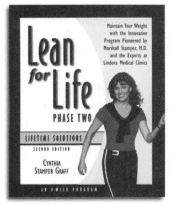

LEAN FOR LIFE PHASE TWO: LIFETIME SOLUTIONS
by Cynthia Stamper Graff

You've lost the weight. How will you keep it off? Maintain your weight with the innovative program pioneered by Marshall Stamper, M.D. and the experts at Lindora Medical Clinics. Based on more than 30 years experience, this book guides you day-by-day through an innovative eight-week program created to help you achieve a state of metabolic equilibrium. Enjoy improved health and enhanced self-esteem as you learn to Eat Better, Move More, and Stress Less.

bodyPRIDE
by Cynthia Stamper Graff
with Janet Eastman & Mark C. Smith

Being a teenager can be tough, especially when you're feeling different or alone. *bodyPride* offers a motivational action plan for teens seeking self-esteem and building better bodies. This book features a 28-day clinically-tested diet plan that's safe and easy for teens. *bodyPride* is an interactive plan that supports young people in going for what they want and feeling better about what they have.

ABOUT THE AUTHOR

Cynthia Stamper Graff is president and CEO of Lindora, Inc., which manages one of the largest medical weight control programs in the United States. A nationally recognized expert in the field of weight management, she has been actively involved in the growth and development of Lindora since 1988. Graff, a leader in integrating technology into the treatment of obesity, has been instrumental in developing Lindora's atHome, atWork and online versions of the Lean for Life program. For three consecutive years, Lindora has been ranked one of the "Top 500 Women Owned Businesses in America" by *Working Woman* magazine.

Graff is the author of *Lean for Life Phase One: Weight Loss* (with Jerry Holderman), *Lean for Life Phase Two: Lifetime Solutions*, and *bodyPRIDE* (with Janet Eastman and Marc C. Smith). She is also the founder of the Lean for Life Foundation, a nonprofit organization that promotes obesity research and educational programs, and funds weight control services to selected low-income, morbidly obese men, women, and children.

An *Orange County Business Journal Women In Business* award winner, Graff is a national Ernst and Young Entrepreneur of the Year Award nominee. She has been a member of the Young Presidents Organization since 1993 and a member of Adaptive Business Leaders since 1998.

Graff holds a law degree from York University in Toronto. She resides in Newport Beach, California.